Effective Clinical Practice

Edited by

Andrew Miles
Myriam Lugon

**Blackwell
Science**

© 1996 by
Blackwell Science Ltd
Editorial Offices:
Osney Mead, Oxford OX2 0EL
25 John Street, London WC1N 2BL
23 Ainslie Place, Edinburgh EH3 6AJ
238 Main Street, Cambridge
  Massachusetts 02142, USA
54 University Street, Carlton
  Victoria 3053, Australia

Other Editorial Offices:
Arnette Blackwell SA
  224, Boulevard Saint Germain
  75007 Paris, France

Blackwell Wissenschafts-Verlag GmbH
  Kurfürstendamm 57
  10707 Berlin, Germany

  Zehetnergasse 6
  A-1140 Wien
  Austria

First published 1996

Set in 10 on 12pt Palatino
by DP Photosetting, Aylesbury, Bucks
Printed and bound in Great Britain
by Hartnolls Ltd, Bodmin, Cornwall

The Blackwell Science logo is a trade mark of
Blackwell Science Ltd, registered at the United
Kingdom Trade Marks Registry

DISTRIBUTORS

Marston Book Services Ltd
PO Box 269
Abingdon
Oxon OX14 4YN
(*Orders:* Tel: 01235 465500
         Fax: 01235 465555)

USA
Blackwell Science, Inc.
238 Main Street
Cambridge, MA 02142
(*Orders:* Tel: 800 215-1000
             617 876-7000
         Fax: 617 492-5263)

Canada
Copp Clark Professional
200 Adelaide Street, West, 3rd Floor
Toronto, Ontario M5H 1W7
(*Orders:* Tel: 416 597-1616
             800 815-9417
         Fax: 416 597-1617)

Australia
Blackwell Science Pty Ltd
54 University Street
Carlton, Victoria 3053
(*Orders:* Tel: 03 9347-0300
         Fax: 03 9347-5001)

A catalogue record for this title
is available from the British Library

ISBN 0-632-03908-6

1002706151

Contents

Preface

Review of the literature in health services research and public health medicine that has accumulated since the promulgation of the NHS reforms of 1989 bears witness to the evolution of an ideological dogma: *clinical guidelines derived from scientific evidence can be implemented through audit into routine clinical practice producing measurable increases in the quality of care delivered to patients and measurable decreases in the cost ineffectiveness of healthcare services.*

A systematic approach to the evaluation and analysis of the key components of this dogma was, we felt, urgently necessary, with several questions needing to be posed. *Scientific evidence:* Where from? How synthesised? Of what grade? *Clinical guidelines:* How constructed? On what evidence? How generalisable to individual patients? Of what medico-legal significance? *Guideline introduction into routine practice through audit:* With what methodology? How will identified divergences from 'recommended' practice be judged as applications of clinical judgement or demonstrations of medical rebellion? Can and should healthcare purchasing influence this process? *Measurable increases in the quality of care:* How will 'quality' be defined? How will it be measured in a statistically sound, clinically valid manner? Can it be purchased by healthcare commissioners? *Measurable decreases in the cost ineffectiveness of healthcare services:* Can such decreases be expected in the face of new technologies and drugs of proven efficacy yet high cost? How can clinicians be assured that successful cost containment exercises are not associated – in the politically unpalatable longer term – with decreases in the quality of care and acceptability of clinical outcome? *Care delivered to patients:* What are patients' expectations of clinical audit and the evidence-based healthcare movement? How can patients influence the quality and cost of their care?

It was in search of the answers to these pivotal questions that led us to commission the individual chapters which constitute the current volume. We have aimed to be sufficiently comprehensive, providing material of immediate use to colleagues actively working within the fields of clinical practice evaluation and health services research. At the same time, we have been concerned to provide adequate background and history to enable teachers and students in these fields to produce, respectively, their lectures and coursework.

We believe that this volume will stimulate contention and debate within the particular subject areas of the individual chapters and that, as a consequence, we will have contributed significantly to the growing science of health services research and therefore to the development of modern health services. We recommend *Effective Clinical Practice* to all medical and clinical colleagues, to health scientists and academics, to managers and to all students of the health sciences.

Professor Andrew Miles
Dr Myriam Lugon

List of Contributors

Jonathan Asbridge RGN, DipN
Nursing Director, Oxford Radcliffe Hospital NHS Trust, Oxford.

Paul Bentley MB ChB, PhD, FRCP, FRCPath
Consultant Haematologist and formerly Medical Director, Llandough Hospital, Cardiff.

David Bowden MA, FHSM, FRSA
Chief Executive, Merrett Health Risk Management Ltd, Brighton and formerly District General Manager, Brighton Health Authority, Brighton.

Nick Freemantle BA (Hons), MA
Senior Research Fellow, Centre for Health Economics and Department of Health Sciences and Clinical Evaluation, University of York.

Joseph Grey BSc (Hons), MB BCh, PhD, MRCP
Senior Registrar, Department of Medicine for the Elderly, University Hospital of Wales, Cardiff.

Andrew Haines MD, FRCGP, FFPHM, FRCP
Professor of Primary Healthcare, Department of Primary Healthcare and Population Sciences, Royal Free Hospital School of Medicine, London.

Brian Hurwitz MA, MSc, MD, MRCP, MRCGP
Senior Lecturer in General Practice, Imperial College School of Medicine, London.

Myriam Lugon MD, FRCP
Medical Director and Consultant Physician, Whipps Cross Hospital, Forest Healthcare NHS Trust, London.

Andrew Miles BSc (Hons), MSc, MPhil, PhD
Deputy Director, Centre for the Advancement of Clinical Practice, European Institute of Health and Medical Sciences, University of Surrey and Visiting Professor of Health Services Research, Faculty of Science and Health, University of East London, London.

Declan O'Neill MPH, MFPHM, FAFPHM, FRACMA
Director, Health Improvement, New South Wales Health Department, Sydney, Australia.

Andreas Polychronis MB BCh
Senior House Physician, Department of Medicine for the Elderly, Guy's Hospital, Guy's and St Thomas's Hospitals NHS Trust, London.

Nicholas Price BA (Hons)
Integrated Care Pathways R&D Co-ordinator, Royal Surrey County Hospital and Associate Research Fellow, Centre for the Advancement of Clinical Practice, University of Surrey.

Marianne Rigge BA (Hons)
Director, College of Health, London.

Ian Watt, MSc, MB ChB, MPH, MFPHM
Senior Research Fellow and Honorary Consultant in Public Health Medicine; NHS Centre for Reviews and Dissemination, University of York.

1 ◆ The Development of Quality in Clinical Practice I: Definitions, Applications and Initiatives

Andrew Miles, Myriam Lugon and Andreas Polychronis

Introduction

'So what exactly do the new enthusiasts for "quality" mean by this word? What is this property that they claim should be pursued, managed, directed and above all demonstrated throughout the NHS? Remarkably, while there is widespread agreement that "quality matters", that its presence in the health service is extremely important and even that its absence costs substantial sums of money, there is little agreement over what this thing is that matters so much, nor, in all the "quality" literature, are there any attempted definitions of the central idea that could stand up to serious scrutiny. Instead, the debate about how to achieve quality is phrased in pseudo-intellectual "management-speak", whose quasi-economic ugliness fails to disguise a shocking lack of precision. This language is permeated by platitudinous declarations of deeply held beliefs in, and an absolute dedication to, "total quality". It seems that when one's explanation of a concept is equivocal, unequivocal commitment to it will do as a substitute, so writers testify to their conversion to quality in much the same way that the converts of American evangelists publicly and stridently affirm their faith.'

(Loughlin 1993.)

The word 'quality' has been employed by a diverse range of health professionals in a diverse range of ways. The achievement of 'quality' is the fundamental aim of all of the initiatives which are directed at raising the standards of organisational and clinical practice within health services. Indeed, the achievement and demonstration of 'quality' is the primary objective set for the medical and clinical audit functions. Yet despite the repeated rhetorical emphasis on the need to improve 'quality' within healthcare practices, there is much evidence to suggest that there are fundamental deficiencies in the understanding held by both NHS managers and clinical colleagues of the nature and characteristics of 'quality' in the context of everyday clinical care. This chapter aims to examine the concept of quality, to recommend a

1

working definition and to explore how the audit function – a tool of considerable potential in the development of quality in clinical practice – can be applied in generating academically-tenable, clinically-valid increases in the standards of clinical care delivered to patients.

Quality in healthcare: a conceptual analysis

Loughlin (1993) is clear that to define the word 'quality' is not really to say what it actually refers to. He argues that to define it, we must say what the term means, and states that a good definition helps to explain what the term means to people who do not already know and serves as a guide to future usage, precluding some uses in advance by distinguishing appropriate uses from inappropriate ones. Loughlin continues by showing that if writers employ the term 'quality' to mean 'certain attributes', they are simply confusing two senses of 'quality'. Indeed, he points out that if the qualities of something are simply its attributes then they can, of course, include 'being awful'. However, writers who employ the word 'quality' do so because they wish to describe something as having attributes enabling people to praise it. If the definition is not to be nonsense, he argues, then it must put all emphasis on the word 'important',

> 'in which case it is totally vacuous, for how do we decide which attributes are "important enough to be identified"? If we can decide what is important without appealing to quality, then the notion of quality is irrelevant. If, as some writers claim, the notion of quality is "indispensable", then the "important" characteristics of the service will be the ones that have the "quality", so the definition is circular and empty'

(Loughlin 1993.)

Loughlin believes that attempts to define what quality actually means are rare indeed. He suggests that many writers employ the term 'quality' in persuasive definitions, by which he likens the process to that described by Stevenson (1944). Loughlin argues that persuasive definition is possible because many terms have two elements to their meaning: a descriptive (or factual) element and what Stevenson described as an emotive (or evaluative) element. Stevenson points out that the emotive meaning of a term is invested with a certain force, affecting our attitudes and causing us to approve, or disapprove, of whatever it is applied to. It is therefore capable of affecting our behaviour. The word 'democracy' is utilised as a useful example of a word invested with a particularly strong emotive force. If a government is able to convince the people that it is 'democratic' then it is likely to be accepted by them and people are more likely to acquiesce under its rule than if it is considered to be undemocratic.

Loughlin advances the important point that persuasive definitions are at their most powerful when the descriptive meaning of a term becomes vague and unclear while nevertheless maintaining its emotive force. To define a term persuasively, he argued, is to offer as an 'explanation' of the meaning of an emotive term what is in fact a proposal for revision of that term's descriptive meaning. Loughlin is clear that if defining a term in this way proves successful, then it has accordingly proved possible to persuade the people who hear the definition to accept a revised factual significance for the term. Since the term continues to carry emotive force it has proved disturbingly possible to change their behaviour without their ever understanding that the process has taken place.

Loughlin argues that, just as the word democracy has been subject to persuasive definitions – with its descriptive meaning becoming vague enough for leaders and political systems of radically different types and colours to claim they are all democratic – the term quality has become vaguer still. However, it retains its emotive force to such an extent that no one can possibly disagree that quality is important or that it matters. The defenders of the 'quality revolution' are, Loughlin argues, 'onto a winner,' because by a constant regurgitation of the word quality and its application to given products or practices, a culture is created in which it seems unreasonable to question, criticise or deny that there have been massive improvements since the times before 'quality' was 'rediscovered'. Loughlin wonders how 'so many intelligent people can [have talked] so much nonsense' in relation to the 'quality initiative'.

Formal definitions of 'quality'

In 1988, Brook and Kosecoff (1988) advanced the following formal definition of quality in healthcare:

> 'The performance of specific activities in a manner that either increases or at least prevents the deterioration in health status that would have occurred as a function of a disease or condition. Employing this definition, quality of care consists of two components: *i.* the selection of the right activity or task or contribution of activities, *ii.* the performance of those activities in a manner that produces the best outcome.'

This rather turgid definition was later partnered by a simplified, though rather vague, description by Calman (1992):

> 'Quality is a concept which describes in both quantitative and qualitative terms the level of care or services provided. Quality as a concept therefore has two components. The first is quantitative and measurable, the second is qualitative, though assessable, and associated with value judgements. Quality is a relative not an absolute concept.'

McIntyre (1985) had previously defined quality, though in an interestingly minimalist fashion: 'What is quality? It is the excellence with which a well-defined task is performed.' But he qualified his definition:

'... if you do not know how to define the task you cannot begin to judge whether the performance is excellent. Criteria are very important here. It is not easy to define good care.'

So what should constitute the criteria through which 'good care' and 'quality practice' can be assessed? Probably the most useful definition of clinical quality in this context has been advanced by the Institute of Medicine following extensive research:

'The degree to which health services for individuals and populations increase the likelihood of desired health outcomes and are consistent with current professional knowledge.

(Lohr 1990.)

We believe that the utility of this definition is manifest in the following three components:

(1) 'The degree to which' ... establishes the concept of variability, indicating the potential for measurement through strict quanti- tation and qualitative description of what has been quantified. It is therefore, as Wareham (1994) has pointed out, singularly dis- tinguished from a multiplicity of definitions which discuss 'quality' in idealistic and absolute terms.

(2) 'The likelihood of desired health outcomes' ... represents an explicit recognition that outcomes may be anticipated but not guaranteed and that the relationship between process and out- come is probabilistic and not deterministic.

(3) 'Consistent with current professional knowledge' ... recognises the dependence of the standard of care on the status of scientific knowledge, both that which exists objectively and that held by the individual clinical practitioner.

   Quality management initiatives have proliferated in the NHS as part of the implementation of the NHS reforms. Of those listed in Table 1.1, we focus here on the central role of the clinical audit mechanism in healthcare quality assurance and development.

Clinical audit and the development of quality in clinical practice

The clinical audit function has no small part to play in implementing clinical standards, clinical guidelines and evidence-based medicine into routine care and thus in making effective clinical practice available to patients. Its introduction into health services was not, however, unopposed by the medical profession, though the scale of opposition was not as great, or the concept so intensively debated, as the more prominent components of the NHS reforms. Indeed, consider the

Table 1.1 Quality Initiatives in the National Health Service. Adapted from Taylor (1996).

Initiative/technique	Description
Accreditation systems	Techniques for assessing institutional fitness to practise.
Anticipated recovery pathways	Multi-disciplinary methods for planning and monitoring treatments.
Benchmarking	Comparing processes between competing organisations.
Business process re-engineering	Radical review of organisational activities, implemented using the methods of total quality management.
BS5750/ISO9000	A form of accreditation based on review of documentation of standard operating processes.
Clinical audit	Multidisciplinary, systematic analysis of the quality of patient care.
Cochrane Centre	Part of the NHS research and development programme; it organises systematic reviews of randomised controlled trials and other evidence of the effectiveness of clinical care.
Communications programmes	Good communications between providers of services and all their internal (same organisation) and external customers are an integral part of quality management.
Complaints systems	The facilitation and analysis of customer complaints is important in total quality management.
Consumer surveys	Large numbers of surveys and monitoring exercises, of varying quality, have been conducted by NHS agencies since 1990.
Disease management	Term commonly applied to health care quality management initiatives funded or run by the pharmaceutical industry. Also linked to the US term 'managed care'.
External probity and VFM audit	Includes NHS studies such as those commissioned by the Audit Commission. External audits may have either or both policing and departmental functions
Inspectorates	Public service health and welfare inspectorates include the Health Advisory Service and the Mental Health Commission.
King's Fund organisational audit	A form of accreditation and linked developmental support run by the King's Fund, an independent policy and educational institution.
Patient's Charter	A set of monitored patient rights and standards first established in 1992 as part of central government's Citizen's Charter initiative.

Table 1.1   Continued.

Initiative/technique	Description
Patient Focus	An approach originally developed by US management consultants, designed to ensure that patients' journeys through care processes are timely and convenient.
Performance indicators/targets	As contained, for example, in the Health of the Nation programme.
Protocols/guidelines	Sets of treatment options and agreed decision-making criteria, which may serve as a basis for systematic evaluation of clinical and allied care standards.
Publication initiatives	For example, *Journal of Evaluation in Clinical Practice, Journal of Quality in Health Care, Journal of Evidence-based Medicine, Effectiveness Matters* etc.
Quality of life measurement	There are now over 400 English language instruments available for assessing quality of life, either in relation to specific conditions or overall wellbeing.
Quality management assessment systems	A form of organisational audit. Examples include the Malcolm Baldrige Award in the US and the European Quality Award.
Risk (and claims) management systems	An approach to quality improvement based on techniques designed to minimise the risk of unwanted events for which the organisation might be liable or otherwise incur costs.
Total quality management	TQM techniques seek to enhance organisational sensitivity to customer requirements and optimally involve everyone in an organisation meeting them.

motion carried by 173 votes to 153 at the Annual Representatives meeting of the British Medical Association in 1980:

> 'that this meeting instruct Council and the Chairman of the Representative Body to stop surveying imposed methods of medical audit'.

The motion had centred around the contention that

> 'medical audit could be defined in several ways; all implied an official examination of some or all aspects of the doctors' professional life. This was unnecessary, undesirable and in some ways offensive. Medical audit should be unnecessary because professional activities were so constructed that fair guidelines were already available and adhered to by all but a few doctors. It was unreasonable to inflict audit on the many because of the few who were likely

to be influenced. It was offensive because most doctors were aware of, and proud to shoulder, their professional responsibilities.'

(BMA 1980.)

Indeed, Black (1981) observed:

'There are strong public and parliamentary pressures to bring medical practice under closer scrutiny, whether by the Ombudsman, or in some other way. Some members of the profession maintain that such pressures are to be resisted, without argument and without compromise, and that we should have nothing to do with medical audit, quality control, or whatever.'

The professional sensitivities that precipitated this opposition were derived in part from the recognition that an audit programme would focus attention on the nature of professional practice. This would provide a tool with which excellence could be demonstrated and variation be exposed; a mechanism that would identify medical error and preclude old fashioned and eccentric practices masquerading under the guise of clinical freedom. However, sustained discussion, increased political pressure and an assurance that audit would be educational not punitive led to professional agreement that routine audit of medical practice was appropriate for introduction into the NHS, albeit into a medical culture which supported a self-confirming, self-validating *modus operandi* of clinicians (May 1977) with a profound reluctance to comment on the work of others (McIntyre 1995).

Definitions of audit

An early product of the acceptance of audit as a conceptual ideal was the crystallisation of a definition of audit promulgated within command 666 of the Government White paper, *Working for Patients* (Secretaries of State for Health 1989):

'Medical audit is the systematic, critical analysis of the quality of medical care including the procedures used for diagnosis and treatment, the use of resources and the resulting outcome and quality of life for the patient.'

The definition is highly familiar and has been regurgitated *ad nauseam*, as if repetition of the words 'systematic' and 'critical' was able to imprint those characteristics on what many authors regard to have been an ill-directed, badly-designed audit programme. Some authors have suggested that the definition might be shortened or extended with the general aim of clarifying the nature and purpose of audit.

One purchaser, in a contract with a major provider for clinical audit, has advanced the definition:

'A cyclical activity incorporating both systematic evaluation of clinical practice and action taken in response to the results of this evaluation.'

Difford (1992) has suggested:

> 'examining what we are doing with the aim of making improvements in the care of patients and the use of resources.'

More recently, Nelson (1994) has continued with this minimalism: 'the critical analysis of medical data to improve patients' care'.

Miles *et al.* (1996) have argued that the continuing methodological and philosophical confusion in relation to what audit is and what it should produce, warrants the adoption of a far more focused, rather functional, definition:

> 'that process which results in the availability of quantitative measurements and qualitative descriptions of increased clinical effectiveness and clinical appropriateness of care and similarly measurable increases in the efficiency with which such clinical improvements are delivered to patients'.

The White Paper definition of medical audit has been more recently modified to formulate a definition for clinical audit in recognition of the contribution of nursing and the professions allied to medicine in the structure, process and outcome of patient care. The definition is similarly well recognised:

> 'Clinical audit is the systematic and critical analysis of the quality of clinical care including the procedures used for diagnosis, treatment and care, the associated use of resources and the resulting outcome and quality of life for the patient.'
>
> (Department of Health 1994.)

Clinical audit and professional integrity

Kistemaker (1987) has advanced four professional reasons for commitment to audit based on the need to strive for continued improvement of performance. He argues that a proper level of commitment to audit is quintessentially Hippocratic in nature and that there is a societal necessity since accountability to society is the source of the authority to practise. There is, additionally, an educational necessity since it is vital that familiarity with the increasing technical and administrative complexity of medical practice is maintained so that errors which are costly in terms of human disability or economic loss will be minimised. Finally, Kistemaker argues, there is the necessity for survival and maintenance of professional independence and status since litigation, private-sector competition, short-term contracts, relicensing and NHS internal marketing emphasise the necessity for doctors to demonstrate, in measurable terms, their continuing and increasing proficiency.

The Medical Royal Colleges are fully supportive of the application of the audit function within health services and are actively working to develop its role. The Royal College of Physicians views the teaching of audit principles and practice as 'essential' and is concerned that 'students should see audit in action alongside medical care' (Royal College of Physicians 1993) as part of the critical examination of medical practice. The word critical is, of course, pejorative, but from the perspective of audit needs to be understood clearly as a judgement made by 'Experience and Prudence and Reason and Discourse' (Gale 1667).

Applications of audit within health services

Two formidable obstructions to the application of audit are generally acknowledged to exist within health services:

(1) The cultural status within clinical organisations.

(2) The lack of adequate methodologies through which evidence-based changes can be introduced into routine clinical practice and the resulting benefits to patients quantitatively measured and qualitatively described.

These factors are specifically treated later in this chapter and in the individual chapters which follow. Let us first consider the primary areas for application of audit in health services, such as areas of variation in clinical practice, areas of known susceptibility to medical error, areas of known clinical risk and areas of poor communication such as the primary–secondary care interface.

Clinical audit and the demonstration of variations in clinical practice

Basis for variation in the process and outcome of clinical care
Maynard (1994) has advanced that the practice of medicine and the reform of healthcare systems have a common characteristic – the absence of an adequate scientific base. Clinicians, he says 'when confronted by patients of similar age, sex and condition intervene in different ways'. In advancing such a tenet, Maynard echoes the statement of the Institute of Medicine:

> 'For many clinical conditions and services, the scientific base is limited ... where considerable research has been done and good methods have been applied to analyse it, honest clinicians may come to different conclusions using the same evidence.'
>
> (Field & Lohr 1990.)

As a consequence, medical opinions frequently appear contradictory and variations in clinical practice are now generating increasing concern (Haines & Jones 1994).

In examining variations in clinical practice, Shaw (1989) definitively disagrees with those who hold the contention that medical practice is self-auditing and will therefore be of itself technically, socially and professionally acceptable. Indeed, Shaw points out that objective studies of normal medical practice rarely demonstrate such an assumption to be true. This author reminds us that audit frequently demonstrates the converse to be true and has identified a higher frequency of unacceptable variations in practice and in outcome than anticipated. Indeed, several workers have investigated 'startling variations' (Hopkins 1990) in medical and surgical practice between doctors and between geographical regions (Krakauer *et al.* 1995).

When examples from clinical outcome have been studied, geographical differences in mortality have been identified. Charlton, Silver and Hartley (1983), for example, demonstrated that the mortality associated with conditions generally recognised as amenable to medical intervention was three times higher in some areas of England and Wales than in others. In an important study, Charlton and Lakhani (1986) reported that in the age range 5–64 years, the mortality risk associated with hernia, gallstones and appendicitis varied tenfold between district health authorities in England and Wales, a wide variation that was similarly noted in deaths among people aged 5–44 years from asthma.

Saunders *et al.* (1989) have reported wide variations in the rates at which surgical procedures are performed. They observed a two-fold variation in the tonsillectomy rate between two adjacent small areas in Scotland and demonstrated that a child in Oxford, Wessex or South West Thames region was twice as likely to undergo surgery for glue ear as a child in Trent or South Western region. These authors observed similar variations in surgery rate elsewhere. In Oxfordshire, for example, the hysterectomy rate varied three-fold between general practices and five-fold differences in cardiac surgery rates were observed between English regions. Major differences in surgery rates were also reported for Caesarian section, cataract extraction and for a gamut of other surgical procedures and hospital admissions.

On the basis of these and other findings, Shaw (1989) is convinced that although population risk will be related to the incidence of these conditions, the variation in outcome implies definitive differences in the technical effectiveness of medical care. Hopkins (1990) is in agreement with this, and while agreeing that some variation in practice will be generated by differing patients' needs, believes that such a variation will be small.

Practice variations and the 'styling' of individual clinical practice
The wide variations identified in clinical practice are highly likely to be causally related to difference in 'style' of practice, quite independent of the objective appropriateness of intervention. The investigation of reasons for such differences is professionally and morally necessary and points unequivocally to the need for an effective tool with which to conduct such investigations. Audit, in characterising the nature and extent of variations in the process and outcome of care, enables a comparison and contrast of local modes of practice with objective clinical standards, guidelines and scientific evidence. It thus provides a

basis for agreeing changes in practice that will narrow the discrepancy between the two. The introduction of such changes and the measurement of resulting benefits to patients, may then be undertaken using further advanced audit methodologies, as described in Chapters 3 and 4 of this volume.

Clinical audit in the investigation, demonstration and correction of clinical error

Serious mistakes can occur in clinical practice. It is therefore important that they are recognised and that mechanisms are put in place to prevent their recurrence (McIntyre 1995).

Definition of clinical error

Leape (1994) defines effort as 'an unintended act (either of omission or commission) or one that does not achieve its intended outcome' and points to an accumulating body of evidence which demonstrates that a substantial number of patients are subject to medical error, particularly during the hospital stay. (Leape *et al.* 1991; Leape 1994.)

Clinical error in routine practice

The existence of a significant level of medical error in everyday practice has been recognised for some time. A publication in the *Annals of Internal Medicine* in 1964 documented the fact that 20% of in-patients admitted to a university teaching hospital had demonstrated iatrogenic injury, with 20% of that percentage proving either fatal or warranting the description of 'serious' (Schimmel 1964). Essentially similar data have been reported by independent investigators. Steel *et al.* (1981) have documented the occurrence of an iatrogenic event in 36% of patients admitted to a university teaching hospital, of which 25% of that percentage were labelled 'serious' or 'life-threatening' and the iatrogenic event being related to pharmacotherapy in over half of the cases identified. More recently, Bedell *et al.* (1991) documented 64% of cardiac arrests in one teaching hospital as preventable, with pharmacotherapy being similarly associated with the cardiac event.

Other investigators provide confirmatory observations. Leape (1994) and his colleagues (Leape *et al.* 1991; Brennan *et al.* 1991) have reported similarly distressing observations from a population-based investigation of iatrogenic injury in American hospital in-patients. They discovered that, in New York State, 4% of patients were reported as having sustained an injury that resulted either in prolongation of length of stay or in the manifestation of measurable disability. Leape (1994) points out that for New York State that was equivalent, in 1984 (the year of sampling), to 98 609 patients. Fourteen per cent of those adverse events were found to have proved fatal. Leape points out that if those rates could be considered as typical across the United States, simple extrapolation indicates that 180 000 patients per year die in association with iatrogenic injury. Leape presents this statistic in a painfully tangible manner by reminding us that this is the likely mortality that would result from three jumbo jet crashes every two days.

Awareness and perception of clinical error

It may seem extraordinary that such startlingly high rates of error have escaped the attention of the public and the clinical profession. As Leape (1994) points out:

> 'One reason may be a lack of awareness of the severity of the problem. Hospital-acquired injuries are not reported in the newspapers like jumbo jet crashes, for the simple reason that they occur one at a time in 5000 different locations across (the USA). Although error rates are substantial, serious injuries due to errors are not part of the everyday experience of physicians or nurses, but are perceived as isolated and unusual events...'

Iatrogenic injuries derive principally from clinical error and are thus potentially preventable, but as Leape points out, it is equally important to recognise that iatrogenic injuries are highly likely to represent only a very small percentage of the total number of error events simply because the majority of errors fail to result in injury to the patient. Take, for example, errors related to medication, which several authors have demonstrated as occurring in 2–14% of hospital in-patients (see Leape (1994) for review), but which are not necessarily associated with manifestation of measurable injury.

The role of audit

Audit is an invaluable tool in the demonstration and investigation of medical error and a prominent means by which strategies for error minimisation can be developed and their effectiveness tested. In characterising local clinical practice, audit can identify error, yield data which show the nature and derivation of error, and provide the basis on which organisational and educational changes aimed at error minimisation and preclusion can be agreed. Advanced audit methodologies, such as those described in Chapters 3 and 4 of this volume, may then be employed in monitoring the introduction of these agreed changes into routine care. These can subsequently demonstrate in both quantitative and qualitative terms, the resulting benefits to patients and the organisation. Audit may therefore be employed in the risk management function, as discussed below.

Clinical audit and clinical risk management

It is increasingly clear that non-adherence to so-called best practice standards and failure to extend adequate supervision and training to junior staff are indicative of clinical risk. Clinical audit can therefore play a major role in clinical risk management within NHS provider organisations.

Reasons for managing clinical risk

Delaney (1994) has pointed out that UK government statistics, released in March 1994 in response to a parliamentary question, showed that the number of claims for medical negligence against the NHS exceeds 1600 per year. The cost of failure to address the need for proper clinical risk management with appropriate tools, one of which is clinical audit, has been estimated at £100 million per annum (Knowles 1995). Current thinking increasingly acknowledges that management of clinical risk extends beyond medical practice alone, to the whole range of hospital staff with clinical and managerial responsibilities, and emphasises the need to recognise clinical risk management as a vital component of everyday practice. The increased importance of clinical risk management within the NHS can be directly linked to the loss of Crown Privilege and to the consequent personal liability of chief officers for breaches of legislation and the responsibility of Trusts to fund their own medical negligence claims.

Knowles has identified three principal reasons for managing clinical risk:

- financial reasons
- legal reasons
- moral reasons

From the clinical perspective, the last reason is to be considered of pre-eminent importance, although it is impossible to avoid due consideration of the financial and legal reasons for clinical risk management. Insufficient consideration in operational practice can compromise the ability of the provider institution to exercise its primary function in dispensing effective healthcare in an appropriate and efficient manner.

Specialties and hospital areas associated with high clinical risk

Knowles (1995) identifies the specialty of obstetrics as associated with the highest clinical risk, with other surgical specialties being associated with medium risk and all other specialties associated with low risk. The hospital areas of highest risk are identified by Knowles as delivery rooms, operating theatres and accident and emergency departments. It is therefore of essential importance that effective audit methodologies are employed in characterising local clinical practice within high risk specialties being practised within high risk areas of NHS Trusts. Where audit demonstrates irregularities of a clinical nature (e.g. non-adherence to established 'good practice') or of an organisational nature (e.g. unsafe equipment), changes may be agreed aimed at correcting identified irregularities and deficiencies, and implementing the changes into routine practice monitored by further, advanced audit methods (see Chapters 3 and 4). Such corrections may then be expressed in both quantitative and qualitative terms.

Common principles

Roche (1993) is clear that:

'medical audit and risk management ... have a common purpose –
the enhancement of the quality of care – and operate in similar ways.
A closer and more effective integration of these two processes is
mutually beneficial and may expedite improvement in the standards
of healthcare provision'.

This author has pointed out that clinical audit and clinical risk management programmes share common principles, particularly the use of
adverse effects monitoring and the development of guidelines and
protocols. The author points out that in a surgical specialty, an adverse
events monitoring process would be concerned with incidents such as
high perioperative mortality and, for further example, unplanned
returns to theatre related to post-operative complications. The results
of such an exercise are important to clinicians for audit purposes and to
managers for clinical risk management purposes, given the potential
for litigation. The importance of effective dialogue between clinicians
and managers and the need for a mutually inclusive relationship is
seen to be particularly essential in this context. Knowles (1995), writing
in the *British Journal of Hospital Medicine*, concludes:

'managing clinical risk is not an esoteric interest for a dedicated few,
it is a part of the professional responsibility of every practitioner'.

Vincent (1996) provides the most authoritative recent discourse in this
area.

Primary–secondary interface

The effects of acute clinical intervention in the hospital setting represent only one aspect of the patient episode. Investigations aimed at
assessing the long-term outcome of clinical intervention are gaining
increasing importance in parallel with a concern to view the patient
episode as a whole and to provide continuity of care. This requires
adequate communication between the primary and secondary
healthcare settings and therefore a bridging of the gap, more technically termed the primary–secondary interface.

A specific definition for interface audit is not generally available
(Baker 1994) although it is clear that the term is employed with specific
reference to interaction between clinicians of varying professions
working in the hospital and community settings. Baker has described
methodologies so far applied in this context as essentially ineffective
and of the 'bad apple' variety, with little evidence that the basic principles of audit and total quality management have been properly
understood. This author is clear that interface audit will require a high
degree of cooperation and teamwork, but is unclear as to whether audit
can be productively employed in fostering such a relationship. We
believe that audit is of definitive utility in this context and is in urgent
need of implementation at the primary–secondary care interface in
order to address a multiplicity of well-recognised deficiencies.

A principal concern of clinicians working in community and hospital settings is the lack of adequate communication between them. Writing in the *British Medical Journal*, Jacobs and Pringle (1990) documented only a 40% sufficiency of answers to questions addressed in referral letters to orthopaedic surgeons, though this result needs to take into account the surgeon's judgement of whether or not the questions asked seemed relevant. Inadequate communication across the interface negates attempts to facilitate continuity of care and interferes with the ability to characterise the long-term clinical outcome from acute hospital interventions.

Relevant to the correction of the well-recognised communication deficiencies between the primary and secondary care settings is the respective organisational cultures within each setting. Sulke *et al.* (1991) despaired of the poor nature of the consultant–GP relationship, manifested all too familiarly in the traditional lack of understanding of each other's work (Sibbald *et al.* 1992) and in markedly differing viewpoints on such pivotal issues as appropriateness of referral (Dowie 1983).

Clinical audit has a central role to play in the correction of many of these deficiencies in communication between the primary and secondary healthcare settings. Through use of proper methodologies (see Chapters 3 and 4), this technique may be employed in characterising local clinical and organisational practices in terms of their effectiveness, efficiency and appropriateness, thus demonstrating the status quo and identifying deficiencies. Following such a characterisation, changes based on research evidence and local consensus can be agreed, and their implementation into practice monitored by continuing use of audit methodologies. The subsequent effects of change implementation, in terms of its benefit to patients and the organisation, can then be estimated both quantitatively and qualitatively.

Conclusion

The achievement of quality in clinical practice is proven by its demonstration and measurement, both of which presuppose an understanding of the nature and characteristics of that being demonstrated and measured. It is therefore vital to ensure that all colleagues have a proper understanding of the meaning of the words they employ when talking of quality in health services. Writing which aims to produce such a proper understanding must steer carefully between too vacuous an explanation on the one hand and too complex an explanation on the other. In this chapter we have aimed to steer the middle ground through simple argument and clarification of definitions. Our discussion of four primary areas for application of clinical audit in the development of quality in clinical practice is deliberately theoretical and aimed at demonstrating the potential of the audit function in bringing about measurable improvements in well-defined areas of deficiency and suboptimal performance in health services. Theory is of limited utility until it is employed in informing practice. In Chapter 2 we therefore consider how the standards of care so integral to the audit process are derived, with additional consideration of the methods through which they may be introduced into practice. Chapters 3 and 4 then present and discuss an analytical methodology for routine audit of clinical practice in NHS provider organisations.

References

Baker, R. (1994) What is interface audit? *Journal of the Royal Society of Medicine* **87**: 228–31.

Bedell, S.E., Deitz, D.C., Leeman, D. & Delbanco, T.L. (1991) Incidence and characteristics of preventable iatrogenic cardiac arrests. *Journal of the American Medical Association* **265**: 2815–20.

Black, D. (1981) Apples of discord. *Journal of the Royal Society of Medicine* **74**: 92–100.

BMA (1980) Annual Representatives Meeting. *British Medical Journal* **281**: 325.

Brennan, T.A., Leape, L.L. & Laird, N. (1991) Incidence of adverse effects and negligence in hospitalised patients: results of the Harvard Medical Practice Study – 1. *New England Journal of Medicine* **324**: 370–76.

Brook, R.H. & Kosecoff, J.B. (1988) Commentary: competition and quality. *Health Affairs* **7**: 150–61.

Calman, K. (1992) Quality: a view from the centre. *Quality in Health Care* **1** (Suppl): S28–S33.

Charlton, J.R.H. & Lakhani, A. (1986) *Avoidable deaths study. Birmingham interauthority comparisons.* South Birmingham Health Authority.

Charlton, J.R.H., Silver, R.M. & Hartley, R.M. (1983) Geographical variation in mortality from conditions amenable to medical intervention in England and Wales. *Lancet* **i**: 691–6.

Delaney, L. (1994) Health care law. *Health Care Analysis* **2**: 319–25.

Department of Health (1994) *Clinical Audit: Meeting and Improving Standards in Health Care*, HMSO, London.

Difford, F. (1992) Defining essential data for audit in general practice. In: *Audit in Action*, (ed. R. Smith). BMJ Press, London, pp. 25–33.

Dowie, R. (1983) *General Practitioners and Consultants. A Study of Outpatients Referrals*, King's Fund, London.

Field, M. & Lohr, K. (1990) *Clinical Practice Guidelines: Directions for a New Programme.* National Academy Press, Washington, DC.

Gale, T. (1667) *The Court of the Gentiles, Oxford and London 1667*, Part III, Book 1, Chapter 4, p. 87.

Haines, A. & Jones, R. (1994) Implementing findings of research. *British Medical Journal* **308**: 1488–92.

Hopkins, A. (1989) *Appropriate Investigation and Treatment in Clinical Practice*, Royal College of Physicians, London.

Hopkins, A. (1990) *Measuring the Quality of Medical Care*, Royal College of Physicians, London.

Jacobs, L.G.H. & Pringle, M.A. (1990) Referral letters and replies from orthopaedic departments: opportunities missed. *British Medical Journal* **301**: 470–73.

Kistemaker, W.J.D. (1987) Peer review in the hospitals of the Netherlands. *Austrian Clinical Reviews* **March**: 16–20.

Knowles, D. (1995) Clinical risk management. *British Journal of Hospital Medicine* **53**: 291–2.

Krakauer, H., Bailey Clifton, R., Cooper, H., Yu, W., Skellan, K.J. & Kattak-kuzhy, G. (1995) The systematic assessment of variations in medical practices and their outcomes. *Public Health Reports* **110**: 2–12.

Leape, L.L. (1994) Error in medicine. *Journal of the American Medical Association* **272**: 1851–7.

Leape, L.L., Brennan, T.A. & Laird, N. (1991) The nature of adverse effects and negligence in hospitalized patients: results of the Harvard Medical Practice Study – 2. *New England Journal of Medicine* **324**: 377–84.

Lohr, K. (1990) *Medicare: A Strategy for Quality Assurance*, Institute of Medicine, National Academy Press, Washington, DC.

Loughlin, M. (1993) The illusion of quality. *Health Care Analysis* **1**: 69–73.

May, W.F. (1977) Code and covenant or philanthropy and contract. In: *Ethics in Medicine: Historical Perspectives and Contemporary Concerns*, (eds S.J. Reiser, A.J. Dyck & W.J. Curran), pp. 65–76. MIT Press, Cambridge, MA.

Maynard, A. (1994) Management of medicine. *Medical Audit News* **4**: 140.

McIntyre, N. (1985) Fostering the critical attitude in medicine. *Australian Clinical Review*, September 1985, pp. 139–43.

McIntyre, N. (1995) Evaluation in clinical practice: problems, precedents and principles. *Journal of Evaluation in Clinical Practice* **1**: 5–13.

Miles, A. (1995) Clinical audit: going against the grain? *Audit in General Practice* **3**: 6.

Miles, A., Bentley, D.P., Polychronis, A., Price, N. & Grey, J. (1996) Clinical audit in the National Health Service: fact or fiction? *Journal of Evaluation in Clinical Practice* **2**: 29–35.

Nelson, E.A.S. (1994) Standardised programme for medical audit is needed. *British Medical Journal* **309**: 672.

Roche, M. (1993) Linking medical audit with risk management. *Auditorium* **2**: (Suppl.) 14–15.

Royal College of Physicians (1993) *Medical Audit: A Second Report*, Royal College of Physicians, London.

Saunders, D., Coulter, A. and McPherson, K. (1989) *Variations in Hospital Admission Rates: A Review of the Literature*, King's Fund Project Paper No. 79, King's Fund, London.

Schimmel, E.M. (1964) The hazards of hospitalisation. *Annals of Internal Medicine* **60**: 100–110.

Secretaries of State for Health (1989) *Working for Patients*, Presented to Parliament by Command of Her Majesty, HMSO London.

Shaw, C. (1989) *Medical Audit: A Hospital Handbook*, King's Fund Centre, KFC 89/11, London.

Sibbald, B., Wilkio, P., Raftery, J., Anderson, S. & Freeling, P. (1992) Prescribing at hospital–general practitioner interface II Impact of hospital outpatient dispensing policies in England on general practitioners and hospital consultants. *British Medical Journal* **304**: 31–4.

Steel, K., Gertman, P.M. & Crescenzi, C. (1981) Iatrogenic illness on a general medical service at a university hospital. *New England Journal of Medicine* **304**: 638–42.

Stevenson, C.L. (1944) *Ethics and Language*, Oxford University Press, Oxford.

Sulke, A.N., Paul, V.E., Taylor, C.J., Roberts, R.H. & Norris, A.D.C. (1991) Open access exercise electrocardiography: a service to improve management of ischaemic heart disease by general practitioners. *Journal of the Royal Society of Medicine* **84**: 590–94.

Taylor, D. (1996) Quality and professionalism in health care: an overview of current initiatives in the NHS. *British Medical Journal* **312**: 626–9.

Vincent, C. (1996) *Clinical Risk Management,* BMJ Press, London.

Wareham, N.J. (1994) External monitoring of quality of health care in the United States. *Quality in Health Care* **3**: 97–101.

2 ◆ The Development of Quality in Clinical Practice II: The Derivation and Implementation of Clinical Standards, Guidelines and Research Evidence

Andrew Miles, Myriam Lugon and
Andreas Polychronis

Introduction

'When I was a clinician I was fairly horrified to find out about four years after I qualified that I was actually killing my patients by using a technique which I had been advised to use in medical school. That was an extremely sobering experience: when you take on trust what your teachers have been telling you and you find through trying to apply it that your patients are suffering and dying unnecessarily. I imagine that most of the doctors here have been upset at some stage in their careers to find something which they really believed in because they had read it in a textbook turned out not only not to be useful, but actually harmful. Once you have had that experience, you start to ask questions about where the information being delivered to us as practitioners comes from... As you saw from the Antman Study – which has been copied for you and presented in part by Trevor Sheldon: *because reviewers have not used scientific methods, advice on some lifesaving therapies has been delayed for more than a decade while other treatments have been recommended long after controlled research has shown them to be harmful.* These researchers looked at American textbooks and review articles; but here is one from my own home town, published in 1987. The statement that *the clinical benefits of thrombolysis whether expressed as improved patient survival or preservation of left ventricular function remain to be established* is lethal. [The sentence quoted is 'lethal' only in the sense that it might discourage practitioners from administering thrombolysis, the clinical benefits of which were in fact established in 1983 – Editors.] I think the 2nd Edition of the Oxford Textbook of Medicine has sold about 50 000 or 60 000 copies. Goodness knows how many hundreds of thousands of people have read that information but that is what is available to us. When members of the public are exposed to the new phenomenon called evidence-based health care, they find it astonishing that we health professionals have let our house get into such a muddle... When Archie Cochrane was a medical officer in a prisoner of war camp, he received a leaflet urging him to defend his clinical freedom. His comment was that he would have willingly traded some of his clinical freedom for some reliable information about how to treat his patients... The Cochrane Centre had as its opening statement Archie Cochrane's criticism that the medical profession's house was not in order. He could have applied it equally to nursing, to physiotherapy or to speech therapy. All of the health professionals are in a similar mess...'

(I. Chalmers and T. Sheldon, reported in the House of Lords 1995.)

So spoke Drs Chalmers and Sheldon in evidence given to the House of Lords in January 1995. The evidence presented to Their Lordships ran into some 15 pages of printed Hansard text and was later sensationally reported to the public by the press (Lightfoot & Rogers 1995; Stuttaford 1995). Few colleagues would have felt comfortable in articulating these concerns so spectacularly, but the example given well illustrates the extraordinary delays that can occur between the discovery of an unequivocally effective treatment and its introduction into routine clinical care. Indeed, there is a history in medicine of extraordinary delays between the discovery of unequivocally effective treatments and their introduction into routine clinical practice and further examples are presented in Chapter 5 of this volume.

The reasons which underly these well-documented delays in research implementation are multiple and complex and are the subject of substantial ongoing investigation. In parallel with this work, efforts have been made to design means by which routine clinical practice can be brought more closely in alignment with so-called evidence-based practice. Such initiatives are prominently represented by the development of clinical standards and, particularly, clinical practice guidelines. Such aids to practice demonstrate considerable potential in the development of quality in clinical practice, and their nature and characteristics are examined in detail in this chapter.

Clinical practice protocols, guidelines and standards

The rate at which the term 'guideline' or 'protocol' has appeared in clinical articles during the last ten years has shown a ten-fold increase (Hurwitz 1994), but the enthusiasm leading to such a proliferation has not been matched in terms of implementation. The same is true within the USA where some 20 000 healthcare standards and clinical practice guidelines have been generated by some 500 organisations (Leone 1993; Hurwitz 1994). Despite considerable impetus and enthusiasm in some areas of medicine, the utility of clinical guidelines remains a matter of very considerable debate and represents a source of no small anxiety (Delamothe 1993, Hart 1993). Indeed, they have been seen as:

'... the salvation from the wide variations in medical care and simultaneously lamented as harbingers of the ruination of Medicine as we know it ... those who are fearful focus on the hazards of navigating between the Charybdis of proliferating guidelines and the Scylla of third-party payers and lawyers ready to use the rules against them.'

(Dans 1994.)

Such polarisation of opinion and expression of concern in relation to the medico–legal significance of guidelines and their implication for the exercise of clinical judgement is paralleled in the UK, but the same author is surely persuasive in emphasising that:

'we need to keep them in perspective, they are neither saviours nor villains, just imperfect attempts to care for patients better. Their development can act as beacons into the still vast scientific unknown.'

(Dans 1994.)

The manner in which indications for evidence-based changes in clinical practices are described is of no small importance. Indeed, many doctors interpret the word 'protocol' as unduly restrictive (Hart 1993). However, as Onion and Whalley (1995) point out, the word 'recommendation' 'lacks conviction' and 'policy' has a 'history of being incorporated into doctors' contractual obligations'. For this reason, these authors argue, the description 'clinical guidelines' is to be preferred. Dickinson (1995) feels that the phrase 'clinical guidelines' may have a 'negative ring', invoking images of 'medical cookbooks' in clinicians' minds. This author suggests that a new description, such as 'expert practice support' may be useful.

Let us first examine the characteristics of clinical standards and guidelines before proceeding to examine the methods through which the evidence on which clinical practice guidelines are based is derived.

General characteristics of clinical practice guidelines

When one compares Irvine and Donaldson's (1994) definition of clinical standards with the Institute of Medicine's (1992) definition of clinical guidelines, similarities are immediately apparent. Clinical standards may be defined as

'complex aggregations of criteria built up into a series of statements describing good clinical practice.'

(Irvine and Donaldson 1994.)

Clinical guidelines may be defined as

'systematically developed statements to assist practitioner and patient decisions about appropriate healthcare for specific clinical circumstances.'

(Institute of Medicine 1992.)

Both are aimed at ensuring the efficiency, effectiveness and appropriateness of healthcare intervention and both may be generated from clinical evidence of varying scientific integrity or through consensus agreement where frank evidence is unavailable.

Levels of flexibility in clinical decision making: clinical standards, guidelines and options

Guidelines consist of statements which describe different aspects of the patient's clinical presentation and on this basis indicate the nature of the intervention which should be considered. Eddy (1990a) is definitive in his categorisation. This author employs the term *standards* to describe interventions which are to be considered appropriate in all circumstances and which therefore preclude flexibility in the individual clinician. The term *guideline* is employed specifically to describe an intervention which affords some degree of flexibility in given clinical circumstances and is therefore to be distinguished from *options* which lack definitive guidance, principally on account of their high level of flexibility. Grimshaw and Russell (1993a, b) prefer the categorisations advanced by Irvine and Donaldson (1994), who describe *mandatory* elements, *near mandatory* elements and *optional* elements.

According to these categorisations, mandatory elements are those components derived from a well-established scientific base and which have an integral relation to a patient's outcome. ISIS-2, for example, demonstrates that early salicylate administration following acute myocardial infarction, in the absence of specific contra-indication, diminishes subsequent mortality (ISIS-2 1988). In circumstances where alternative management strategies exist and where relative effectiveness data are unable, optional practice is possible but relative effectiveness research is automatically indicated.

Deterministic and branching clinical guidelines

Irvine *et al.* (1986) have provided further and useful descriptive terminology. These authors argue that clinical guidelines may be categorised into the broad divisions of *deterministic clinical guidelines* and *branching clinical guidelines*. Deterministic clinical guidelines may be defined as those which consist of a fixed number of elements which are to be followed rigidly. Deterministic clinical guidelines do not admit actions based on deductive medical decision making. As a consequence they have limited applicability in routine clinical practice and are generally more appropriate in situations of acute medical or surgical emergency. Branching guidelines are more commonly known as clinical algorithms or treatment flowcharts and occasionally their guidance will be presented instead in textual format (Margolis *et al.* 1989). Guidelines must demonstrate key characteristics to achieve clinical credibility and these are considered in Chapter 5 of this volume.

The validity of clinical practice guidelines is dependent on the rigour of development

Clinical guidelines must be derived from sound evidence but may, in given circumstances, be supplemented by expert opinion. They should always be considered as 'works in progress' unless supporting data are indisputable, and they remain important mechanisms for discussing with clinicians areas of their practice which do not 'systematically incorporate important advances' (Woolf 1992). The relative validity of the directions provided by clinical guidelines must also depend on the integrity or 'weight' of the scientific evidence on which they are based and which describes the expected clinical outcome (Eddy 1990a–d).

Grimshaw and Russell (1993a) agree that a central factor in guideline integrity and validity is rigorous development based on available scientific evidence. The authors recognise that, in the absence of such a sound scientific base, validity may be conferred by best clinical judgement. Failure to adopt a rigorous approach, they warn, may result in ineffective or even dangerous clinical practice. In reviewing the methods by which evidence may be synthesized, Grimshaw and Russell (1993a) identify five principal techniques:

- expert opinion
- unsystematic literature review
- ungraded systematic review
- graded systematic review
- formal meta-analysis.

Synthesis of evidence: opinion, review and meta-analysis

Expert opinion
Grimshaw and Russell (1993a) point out that in the UK clinical guidelines have been developed by expert groups without a formal review of the literature. Development of clinical guidelines in this way is substantially reliant upon working knowledge of published research in combination with individual clinical experience, in what Grimshaw and Russell (1993a) term 'unevaluative conditions'. It is important to note in this context that as Haynes *et al.* (1983) have pointed out, clinicians' knowledge of published research is frequently incomplete and can be based on misinterpretation of presented results. Guidelines developed in this way may well demonstrate inherent bias and result in perpetuation of opinion-based practice rather than evidence-based practice.

Unsystematic review
Unsystematic review is described by Grimshaw and Russell (1993a) as lacking explicit research strategy, explicit inclusion criteria and formal methods of synthesising evidence. Unsystematic review is in some characteristics superior to guidelines derived by expert opinion in that it expands the evidence base, but is limited somewhat in that important

studies may well be omitted as a consequence of inadequate literature searching. Non-application of appropriate inclusion criteria can generate literature which varies considerably in its overall quality and integrity; selection bias is therefore a prominent and persistent problem of unsystematic review.

Systematic review

The application of definitive search strategies and inclusion criteria, such as minimum levels of acceptability in methodological design of studies, characterises the systematic review. Rigorous methodology is employed to locate and crystallise research data relevant to clinical decision making (Mulrow 1994). Systematic review of clinical intervention is a time-consuming process and often involves substantial international collaboration (Grimshaw *et al.* 1995). The recent collaboration between antiplatelet trialists, for example, involved the aggregation of original patient data on some 130 000 subjects in over 300 randomised controlled trials (Antiplatelet Trialists' Collaboration 1994a–c).

Ungraded systematic reviews, for example, employ explicit standards in judging the scientific validity and clinical utility of published research, ensuring the exclusion of methodologically unsound work. Grimshaw and Russell (1993a) give the example of Haynes *et al.* (1984) who, in reviewing 248 potential studies published between 1970 and 1983 for inclusion in a systematic review of the effectiveness of continuing medical education and using rigorous inclusion criteria, were able to include only seven for final analysis.

Graded systematic review has been described by Sackett (1986) and precludes the exclusion of research from sources other than randomised controlled trials which are the foci of most ungraded systematic reviews. The methodology described by Sackett involves the grading of evidence in which research studies are ranked by design. A large randomised trial with low error risk factors would receive Level 1 ranking, but a series of cases with no control data would receive Level 5 ranking. In this way, guideline developers can grade recommendations for best clinical practice directly according to the integrity of the research data that they have examined. An A-graded practice recommendation would be recognised as one deriving from at least one Level 1 study.

Meta-analysis

Many clinicians will agree that certain clinical guidelines which have been crystallised from systematic reviews of the research literature are appropriate for rapid introduction into routine practice. In other cases, however, the same clinicians will express reservations in relation to the scientific integrity of the evidence on which they are based and the process by which they have been derived. Meta-analysis can represent a powerful technique of considerable utility when contradictory data are generated by trials which have examined essentially similar subjects and where data from several trials require combination. It continues to be promoted as a source of infallible dogma for clinical decision making, but methodological deficiencies in this process remain a source of significant concern (Eysenck 1995; Polychronis *et al.* 1996a, b).

Eysenck (1995) has elegantly articulated the difficulties that warrant serious consideration. A principal concern is in the inclusiveness of meta-analysis, in that meta-analysis can examine data that are 'good, bad, and indifferent'. Smith *et al.* (1980) were among the first to pioneer the technique in an effort to preclude subjectivity in outcome analysis. These investigators reasoned that so-called 'bad' studies (for example, those with deficiencies in study design) are frequently excluded by reviewers from the process of outcome analysis and that such exclusion is made as a result of subjective judgement. The authors rightly pointed out that reviewers will often formulate exclusion/inclusion criteria in order to 'favour a favourite hypothesis or vested ideological interest'. However, their advocacy of comprehensive inclusiveness is inherently problematic in its own right because many articles that have received unfavourable criticism will have received it on objective grounds. Indeed, if a study has simply not employed statistically valid sampling, valid conclusions cannot be drawn from its data. The study's exclusion would therefore be warranted on purely objective grounds.

This has led many authors to ask the question, 'what constitutes a good review?' Agreed, the discovery of subjectivity in any analysis is cause for immediate concern and investigation, but also to be considered are the very relevant factors of what Eysenck (1994) describes as

'... intimate knowledge of the field, the participants, the problems that arise, the reputation of different laboratories, [and] the likely trustworthiness of individual scientists...'

Meta-analysis routinely fails to consider these factors and while precluding one form of subjective bias, it cumulatively aggregates in systematic fashion any inherent biases in the original reports. As Eysenck has pointed out, these biases may or may not balance out.

Eysenck has written previously about these problems (see Eysenck (1995) for discussion) and has recently articulated the principal methodological considerations that should be taken into account when performing or interpreting meta-analyses (Eysenck 1995). These include non-linearity of regressions, multivariate versus univariate effects, restriction of coverage, non-homogeneity of summarised data, grouping of different causal factors resulting in estimates of effects of equivocal meaning and impaired ability to detect discrepancies because of a theory-directed approach. Indeed, Eysenck (1994) concludes that:

'meta-analysis may not be the one best method for studying the diversity of fields for which it has been used'.

Indeed, the author believes that meta-analyses are:

> 'often employed in an effort to recover something from poorly designed studies, studies of insufficient statistical power, studies that give erratic results and those resulting in apparent contradictions'.

Careful investigation can avoid such pitfalls but, in the process of doing so, can often be observed to introduce subjectivity, something which meta-analysis is theoretically designed to avoid. In his textual conclusion, Eysenck provides a sobering thought:

> 'If a medical treatment has an effect so recondite and obscure as to require meta-analysis to establish it, I would not be happy to have it used on me. It would seem better to improve the treatment, and the theory underlying the treatment.'
>
> (Eysenck 1995.)

Clinical acceptability and scientific validity of clinical practice guidelines

Grimshaw and Russell (1993a) emphasise the dependency for validity and acceptability of clinical practice guidelines on the nature and characteristics of the guideline development group. These authors describe three principal categories of guideline development groups: *internal* groups, *intermediate* groups and *external* groups. An internal group is characterised by having as its members the clinicians who will subsequently use the guidelines synthesised. An intermediate group is characterised by the inclusion of representatives of the clinicians who will subsequently use the guidelines produced by the group. An external group is characterised by non-inclusion of the clinicians who will subsequently employ the guidelines developed. It has been stated that guidelines developed by the clinicians who will use them, such as in internal groups, are more likely to be implemented than others, as a consequence of a perception of ownership. Only two studies (Putnam & Curry 1985; North of England Study of Standards and Performance in General Practice 1992) out of four (Sommers *et al.* 1984; Putnam & Curry 1985, 1989; North of England Study of Standards and Performance in General Practice 1992) identified by Grimshaw *et al.* (1995) provided data in support of that contention.

Importance of specialty composition

The specialty composition of internal, intermediate and external guideline development groups has been shown to play an important role in determining the nature of the developed practice guidelines. Differences in the practice guidelines for carotid endarterectomy formulated by a panel made up entirely of surgeons, and another that included surgeons, neurologists and other specialties were illustrated by Leape *et al.* (1992) and similar observations have been reported in relation to practice guidelines for cholecystectomy (Scott and Black 1991).

Potential bias of peer-group, Delphi technique and consensus conference methods

Audet *et al.* (1990) have described three principal methodologies for development of clinical practice guidelines; the peer group method, the Delphi technique method and the consensus conference method. All three methodologies are potentially biased with minimal evidence being available in terms of their relative merits (Grimshaw and Russell 1993a; Russell *et al.* 1994). As a consequence, Grimshaw and Russell (1993a) advise against use of the primary method of development as a classification factor when talking about validity of guideline development and point to the work of Woolf (1992) in characterising four secondary methodologies for clinical practice guideline development which are directly related to the nature of the decision making. They are:

- informal consensus-based guideline development
- formal consensus-based guideline development
- evidence-based guideline development
- explicit guideline development.

Informal consensus
The development of clinical practice guidelines using the informal consensus method is characterised by its use of poorly defined and frequently implicit criteria for decision making. Clinical practice guidelines therefore derive from 'global subjective judgement' (Eddy 1990a–d). The informal consensus method is able to produce clinical guidelines quickly because it is a technique lacking complicated analytical processes, but the guidelines so derived are frequently unaccompanied by methodological information with which to convince clinicians of their validity. Informal consensus has been widely employed within the UK to date (Newton *et al.* 1992).

Formal consensus
The development of clinical practice guidelines using the formal consensus method is characterised by the employment of a far more structured approach than is present in informal consensus. However, it similarly fails to demonstrate an explicit association of practice recommendations with an established evidence base (Woolf 1992).

Evidence-based methods
The development of clinical guidelines using the evidence-based method is characterised by an explicit association of practice recommendations with an established evidence base (Woolf *et al.* 1990). In

circumstances where this evidence base has not been rigorously derived it may be supplemented by expert opinion, though this must be documented.

The explicit method

The explicit guideline method is rarely used to develop clinical practice guidelines. It involves evaluation of the benefits, risks and costs of potential clinical interventions through estimation of the probability and value of each potential outcome, thus formulating a 'balance sheet' to facilitate patient choice (Eddy 1990a–d; Grimshaw and Russell 1993a).

Inquiry into clinical practice guideline derivation and validity

Grimshaw and Russell (1993a) are clear in recommending the use of systematic literature reviews, external guideline development groups constituted by representatives of all key disciplines and the explicit linkage of clinical practice recommendations with an evidence base of established scientific integrity. These authors conducted a systematic review of rigorous evaluations of clinical practice guidelines appearing in the published literature between 1976 and 1992. It is an excellent reference work which has been recently updated by these authors and their associates (Grimshaw *et al.* 1995) to include a further 32 studies which were previously unidentified or published up until June 1994. The authors reviewed investigations of clinical guidelines that were formulated primarily for medical staff if they: employed rigorous study design aimed at evaluating guideline effectiveness in terms of the process of care or clinical outcome for patients; and reported sufficient data for statistical analysis.

A landmark study of clinical practice guideline derivation and validity

Grimshaw *et al.* (1995) identified a total of 91 studies relating to a wide variety of clinical settings and procedures, of which only 14 were UK based. The authors describe 35 studies of clinical care, 34 of preventive care and 22 of prescribing/using radiological or laboratory investigation. Grimshaw *et al.* observed that 81 of the 87 studies which investigated effects on the process of care in terms of guideline adherence reported improvements that were considered significant. Twelve of the seventeen studies which assessed clinical outcome reported similarly significant improvements. The authors reported that each of the 14 studies conducted in the UK demonstrated significant improvements in guideline compliance with a definitive improvement in clinical outcome being observed in one study. When the authors examined evidence from those studies demonstrating the most reliable evidence, 43 out of 44 Grade 1 studies showed significant changes in process, while 8 out of 11 showed significant change in clinical outcome. These are important observations which suggest that rigorously developed clinical practice guidelines can change routine clinical practice and influence the nature of clinical outcome in the patient.

Grey zones of clinical practice and the limitations of 'evidence'

It is important to appreciate that evidence-based medicine is not yet at a point where it can produce an answer to 'all ills' (Polychronis *et al.* 1996a, b). Many individuals and institutions, particularly public ones such as the Government, are characterised by believing that they can and they show inflated expectations. As Naylor (1995), writing in *The Lancet* has pointed out, evidence-based medicine contributes little assistance in the many 'grey zones' of clinical practice, where the evidence in relation to risk–benefit ratios of competing clinical options is incomplete or contradictory. Naylor believes that, almost by definition, this intellectual terrain is poorly charted, although the RAND research demonstrates its considerable potential.

In developing criteria for the assessment of clinical appropriateness, RAND constitutes panels of clinical experts who rate hundreds of hypothetical cases on a risk–benefit scale (Brook *et al.* 1986; Park *et al.* 1989). The research shows that ratings for some clinical scenarios inevitably cluster in the uncertain middle of the scale, and disagreement within the panel results in definitions of appropriateness for other clinical scenarios not being possible. Naylor (1995) has shown that, when ratings of a given nation's experts are applied to charts audited in the same country, there is a notable proportion of 'grey-zone procedures'. Naylor has additionally illustrated how cross-national panellists' ratings can generate differing results when applied to the same data. Indeed, US panels are characterised by being relatively more action-orientated in areas of uncertainty than, for example, UK panels, whilst panels in Canada display intermediate behaviour.

Additional research published by RAND demonstrates that surgeons view surgery with considerably less uncertainty than physicians, and generalists are significantly more conservative than specialists (Leape *et al.* 1992; Fraser *et al.* 1993). Naylor (1995) believes that all of these ratings demonstrate not simply the role of evidence but also the roles of inference and experience. As a consequence, as Scott and Black (1991) point out, panellists may be pooling ignorance as much as distilling wisdom and, as Phelps (1993) has emphasised, the decision roles for equivocality versus inappropriateness are themselves arbitrary. It is similarly clear that, as Lomas *et al.* (1988) have said, if evidence were required from randomised controlled trials in support of each indication, the 'grey zone' would be significantly extended.

Paralytic indecisiveness does not characterise routine clinical practice

Naylor (1995) points out the sobering fact that:

'the boundaries of the grey zones are themselves uncertain, varying with the evidence and its interpretation. Clinical medicine seems to consist of a few things we know, a few things we think we know – but probably don't; and lots of things we don't know at all.'

There are therefore many clinical actions which evidence alone cannot guide and one might therefore expect what Naylor describes as 'paralytic indecisiveness' to be more common in routine clinical practice than it actually seems to be. Many clinicians, however, become accustomed to medical decision making in situations of clinical uncertainty but become confident in this educated guesswork to the point where it is easy to confuse personal opinion with evidence or personal ignorance with genuine scientific uncertainty. In the section of Naylor's (1995) article entitled 'Reconciling the new evaluative sciences and old arts', the author makes the point that clinical guideline writers do not act helpfully if they advance an expert consensus that has failed to distinguish fact from fervour. The author points out that

'if clinical guidelines and other trappings of evidence-based medicine are to be credible, they must distil the best evidence about what ought to be done in practice in ways that honestly acknowledge what we do and do not know about a topic ... more generally, the prudent application of evaluative sciences will affirm rather than obviate the need for the art of medicine'.

Conclusion

The development of quality in clinical practice will depend on a willingness of clinicians to refer increasingly to the accumulated (and accumulating) research evidence in their everyday management of patients. The volume and complexity of data is such that most clinicians within the modern NHS would find such a task practically impossible. In this context, the utility of clinical guidelines is clear, although many practitioners retain significant concern in relation to the nature of the evidence on which guidelines are based and the medico–legal implications of their use. Of additional concern is the potential for obviation of clinical judgement that a radical imposition of guidelines would precipitate. In order to consider the use of clinical guidelines in the decision-making process, clinicians must understand *why* they need to modify their practices and will need to feel confident that the evidence base of recommended guidelines is sound. The role of continuing clinical education in this context seems clear and is examined later in Chapters 3 and 4.

Changes agreed in theoretical principle as a result of knowledge and understanding provided by continuing clinical education do not automatically achieve translation into operational practice. It is in this context that the central role of the audit function becomes clear. Clinical audit represents a powerful operational mechanism through which clinical practice guidelines can be introduced into routine clinical practice. Direct characterisation of local clinical practice through use of the audit process, and direct comparison and contrast of that practice with guideline-directed practice, can stimulate debate aimed at narrowing the discrepancy between the two. When guideline-based changes have been agreed in this way, their introduction into routine practice can be monitored and facilitated through further use of the audit function, with audit proving of ultimate use in characterising the resulting benefits to patients.

The complementarity of clinical research and clinical audit is theoretically explicit in this context. The practical benefits of such symbiosis are only likely to be realised, however, when methodologies for functional integration of the R&D and clinical audit mechanisms are developed, accepted and implemented. This will necessitate a continuing change in the organisational culture which continuing clinical education will have no small place in advancing. When these objectives have been met, measurable increases in the quality of patient care can be expected.

References

Antiplatelet Trialists' Collaboration (1994a) Collaborative overview of randomised controlled trials of antiplatelet therapy I. Prevention of death, myocardial infarction and stroke by prolonged antiplatelet therapy in various categories of patients. *British Medical Journal* **308**: 81–106.

Antiplatelet Trialists' Collaboration (1994b) Collaborative overview of randomised trials of antiplatelet therapy II. Maintenance of vascular graft or arterial patency by antiplatelet therapy. *British Medical Journal* **208**: 159–68.

Antiplatelet Trialists' Collaboration (1994c) Collaborative overview of randomised trials of antiplatelet therapy III. Reductions in venous thrombosis and pulmonary embolism by antiplatelet prophylaxis among surgical and medical patients. *British Medical Journal* **308**: 235–46.

Audet, A.M., Greenfield, S. & Field, M. (1990) Medical practice guidelines: current activities and future directions.

Brook, R.H., Chassin, M.R., Fink, A., Solomon, D.H. & Kosecoff, J.B. (1986) A method for the detailed assessment of the appropriateness of medical technologies. *International Journal of Technological Assessment in Health Care* **2**: 53–64.

Dans, P.E. (1994) Credibility, cookbook medicine, and common sense: guidelines and the college. *Annals of Internal Medicine* **120**: 966–8.

Delamothe, T. (1993) Wanted: guidelines that doctors will follow. *British Medical Journal* **307**: 218.

Dickinson, E. (1995) Using market principles for healthcare development. *Quality in Health Care* **4**: 40–44.

Eddy, D.M. (1990a) Practice policies – what are they? *Journal of the American Medical Association* **263**: 877–80.

Eddy, D.M. (1990b) Clinical decision making: from theory to practice. The challenge. *Journal of the American Medical Association* **263**: 287–90.

Eddy, D.M. (1990c) Practice policies: where do they come from? *Journal of the American Medical Association* **263**: 1265–75.

Eddy, D.M. (1990d) Comparing benefits and harms: the balance sheet. *Journal of the American Medical Association* **263**: 2239–43.

Eysenck, H.J. (1994) Meta-analysis and its problems. *British Medical Journal* **309**: 789–92.

Eysenck, H.J. (1995) Meta-analysis or best-evidence synthesis? *Journal of Evaluation in Clinical Practice* **1**: 29–36.

Fraser, G.M., Pilpel, D., Hollis, S., Kosecoff, J.B. & Brook, R.H. (1993) Indications for cholecystectomy: the results of a consensus panel approach. *Quality Assurance in Health Care* **5**: 75–80.

Grimshaw, J. & Russell, I.T. (1993a) Achieving health gain through clinical guidelines. I: Developing scientifically valid guidelines. *Quality in Healthcare* **2**: 243–8.

Grimshaw, J. & Russell, I.T. (1993b) Effect of clinical guidelines on medical practice: a systematic review of rigorous evaluations. *Lancet* **342**: 1317–22.

Grimshaw, J., Freemantle, N., Wallace, S., Russell, I., Hurwitz, B., Watt, I., Long, A. & Sheldon, T. (1995) Developing and implementing clinical practice guidelines. *Quality in Health Care* **4**: 55–64.

Hart, O. (1993) Protocols or guidelines, or neither? *British Medical Journal* **306**: 816.

Haynes, R.B., Sackett, D.L. & Tugwell, P. (1983) Problems in handling of clinical research evidence by medical practitioners. *Archives of Internal Medicine* **143**: 1971–75.

Haynes, R.B., Roms, D.A., McKibbon, A. & Tugwell, P. (1984) A critical appraisal of the efficacy of continuing medical education. *Journal of the American Medical Association* **251**: 61–4.

House of Lords (1995) *Minutes of Evidence Taken Before the Select Committee on Science and Technology*, Subcommittee 1: Medical Research and the NHS Reforms, Session 1994–1995, 31 January 1995. HMSO, London.

Hurwitz, B. (1994) Clinical guidelines: proliferation and medicolegal significance. *Quality in Health Care* **3**: 37–44.

Institute of Medicine (1992) *Guidelines for Clinical Practice: from Development to Use*. National Academic Press, Washington DC.

Irvine, D. & Donaldson, L. (1994) Quality and standards in healthcare. In: *Quality Assurance in Medical Care* (eds J.S. Beck, I.A.D. Bouchier & I.T. Russell), Royal Society of Edinburgh, Edinburgh.

Irvine, D., Russell, I.T. & Hutchinson, A. (1986) Performance review in general practice. In: *In Pursuit of Quality?* (eds D.A. Pendleton, T.P.C. Schofield & M.L. Marinker), Royal College of General Practitioners, London.

ISIS-2 (1988) Second International Study of Infarct Survival Collaborative Group Randomised trial of intravenous streptokinase, oral aspirin, both, or neither among 17 187 cases of suspected myocardial infarction. *Lancet* **ii**: 349–60.

Leape, L.L., Park, R.G., Kahan, J.P. & Brook, R.H. (1992) Group judgements of appropriateness: the effect of panel composition. *Quality Assurance in Health Care* **4**: 151–9.

Leone, A. (1993) Medical practice guidelines are useful tools in litigation. *Medical, Malpractice, Law and Strategy* **10**: 1–6.

Lightfoot, L. & Rogers, L. (1995) Hundreds killed by doctors relying on outdated manuals. *The Sunday Times*, 5 February 1995, pp. 1 and 2.

Lomas, J., Anderson, G.M., Enkin, M., Vayda, E., Roberts, R. & MacKinnon, B. (1988) The role of evidence in the consensus process. *Journal of the American Medical Association* **259**: 3001–3008.

Margolis, C.Z., Cook, C.D., Barak, N., Adler, A. & Geertsma, A. (1989) Clinical algorithms teach paediatric decision making more effectively than prose. *Medical Care* **27**: 576–92.

Mulrow, C.D. (1994) Rationale for systematic reviews. *British Medical Journal* **309**: 597–9.

Naylor, D.C. (1995) Grey zones of clinical practice: some limits to evidence-based medicine. *Lancet* **345**: 840–42.

Newton, J., Hutchinson, A., Steen, I.N., Russell, I.T. & Haines, E.V. (1992) Educational potential of medical audit: observations from a study of small groups setting standards. *Quality in Healthcare* **1**: 256–9.

North of England Study of Standards and Performance in General Practice (1992) Medical audit in general practice: effects on doctors' clinical behaviour and the health of patients with common childhood conditions. *British Medical Journal* **304**: 1480–88.

Onion, C.W.R. & Walley, T. (1995) Clinical guidelines: development, implementation and effectiveness. *Postgraduate Medical Journal* **71**: 3–9.

Park, R.E., Fink, A. & Brook, R.H. (1989) Physician ratings of appropriate indications for three procedures: theoretical indications vs indications used in practice. *American Journal of Public Health* **79**: 445–7.

Phelps, C.E. (1993) The methodologic foundations of studies of the appropriateness of medical care. *New England Journal of Medicine* **329**: 1241–5.

Polychronis, A., Miles, A. & Bentley, D.P. (1996a) Evidence-based medicine: Reference? Dogma? Neologism? New orthodoxy? *Journal of Evaluation in Clinical Practice* **2**: 1–3.

Polychronis, A., Miles, A. & Bentley, D.P. (1996b) The protagonists of evidence-based medicine: arrogant, seductive and controversial. *Journal of Evaluation in Clinical Practice* **2**: 9–12.

Putnam, R.W. & Curry, L. (1985) Impact of patient care appraisal on physician behaviour in the office setting. *Canadian Medical Association Journal* **132**: 1025–9.

Putnam, R.W. & Curry, L. (1989) Physicians' participation in establishing criteria for hypertension management in the office: will patient outcomes be improved? *Canadian Medical Association Journal* **140**: 806–809.

Russell, I.T., Grimshaw, J.M. & Wilson, B.J. (1994) Epidemiological and statistical issues in quality assurance. In: *Quality Assurance in Medical Care* (eds J.S. Beck, I.A.D. Bouchier & I.T. Russell). Proceedings of the Royal Society of Edinburgh **101B**: 77–103.

Sackett, D.L. (1986) Rules of evidence and clinical recommendations on the use of anti-thrombotic agents. *Chest* **86**: (Suppl) 2–3.

Scott, E.A. & Black, N. (1991) When does consensus exist in expert panels? *Journal of Public Health Medicine* **13**: 35–9.

Smith, M.L., Glass, V.G. & Miller, T.I. (1980) The benefits of psychotherapy. John Hopkins Press, Baltimore, MD.

Sommers, L.S., Sholtz, R. & Shepherd, R.M. (1984) Physician involvement in quality assurance. *Medical Care* **22**:1115–38.

Stuttaford, T. (1995) Are our doctors dangerously out of date? *The Times*, 7 February 1995, p. 17.

Woolf, S.H. (1992) Practice guidelines – a new reality in medicine. II: Methods of developing guidelines. *Archives of Internal Medicine* **152**: 946–52.

Woolf, S.H., Battista, R.N., Anderson, G.M., Logan, A.G. & Wang, E. (1990) Assessing the effectiveness of preventive manoeuvres: analytic principles and systematic methods in reviewing evidence and developing clinical practice recommendations. *Journal of Clinical Epidemiology* **43**: 891–905.

3 ◆ Methods for Auditing the Totality of Patient Care I: Pre-requisite Management Structures and Organisational Innovations

Andrew Miles, Paul Bentley, Nicholas Price, Andreas Polychronis, Joseph Grey and Jonathan Asbridge

Introduction

Writing in *Medical Education*, Fowkes (1982) noted the lack of general agreement within the medical profession on methods of audit, a deficiency previously articulated by Shaw (1980). More recently, a study by Black and Thompson (1993) of consultant and junior medical staff in four London district general hospitals revealed that 'many doctors did not understand how to undertake audit', while major research by both Hopkins (1993; 1994) and Buttery *et al.* (1994) observed a multiplicity of methodological deficiencies in the general approaches to audit adopted by clinicians since the promulgation of the White Paper definition in 1989.

Soundness of methodological approach is fundamental to securing the success of clinical audit within provider organisations and is thus central to the generation of measurable improvements in the quality of clinical care being delivered to patients. It is therefore disturbing that methodological deficiencies may still be observed in general approaches to audit (Buttery *et al.* 1994; Miles *et al.* 1996a, b), with no author yet recommending a formal system for critical inquiry into clinical practice. It was the recognition of the unsatisfactory nature of this situation which led us to develop a system aimed at critical assessment of the quality of care being dispensed within NHS provider organisations.

Critical inquiry into clinical practice

When discussing the rationale underlying the care that they administer and the interventions that they employ, most clinicians will refer to:

- knowledge gained in medical school and during houseman years
- scientific publications in medical journals and
- the concept of clinical judgement itself.

There is clear evidence to show that research findings are inadequately translated into routine clinical practice and that this derives not only from a well-recognised clinical resistance to change, but is attributable also, as pointed out in Chapters 1 and 2, to the lack of well-established methodologies with which evidence-based clinical guidelines can be introduced into routine clinical practice (Haines & Jones 1994).

The quality of clinical care can be markedly enhanced by systematic investigation and critical inquiry into clinical practice. Progress in this context can be assured through more rational use of existing techniques and the accelerated development of new ones. Increases in the quality of clinical practice are also associated with a multi-disciplinary approach to practice development and the replacement of clinical opinion with definitive research evidence. Sound methodologies for clinical audit are fundamental to the translation of such rhetoric into reality.

Organisational innovation

Paxton *et al.* (1993) point out that making audit work – especially clinical or multi-disciplinary audit – is an organisational innovation. It requires substantial numbers of people in different parts of the organisation to do new things, to work together in new ways and to keep on doing so in an area which is intrinsically threatening. Considerations of what will constitute 'effective audit methodology' must therefore include examinations of professionals' concerns as matters quite separate to the basic processes of data capture and statistical analysis.

Walshe and Coles (1993) have emphasised that the understanding of how and why medical audit is (or is not) successful in producing quality improvements is very limited. These authors identified a need to establish the characteristics of good audit practice and to understand the underlying mechanisms of that practice as the basis for improving the audit programme's effectiveness. The structured, evaluative approach required to advance such understanding was undertaken by these authors and their associates with interesting and valuable results (Walshe & Coles 1994a, b; Walshe *et al.* 1994; Buttery *et al.* 1994). These results showed wide variations in the extent and complexity of audit activity, very little comparative information in relation to the use of the audit resource and to which activities actually occurred and to what benefits were produced. Other independent investigators (Hopkins 1993, 1994; Kerrison *et al.* 1993; Buxton 1994) agreed with these findings. Miles *et al.* (1996a, b) insist that these deficiencies, and the consequent spectacular lack of demonstration of clinical benefit from audit, derive from profoundly inadequate methodology, itself in part resulting from a failure to recognise audit as an essentially scientific process.

The need for a scientific approach to clinical audit

Russell and Wilson (1992) were among the first investigators to recognise the scientific nature of audit, describing it as 'the third clinical science, with its own theories, techniques and literature'. Buxton (1994) is similarly clear in describing audit as a 'scientific', but also a 'complex and not easily replicable technology' which, if it is to prove effective, must follow a relatively complicated sequence of processes, involving a difficult set of organisational procedures. Buxton argues that at the present time audit is not *obviously* more beneficial than, for example, a drug of unproven efficacy or a surgical procedure of unproven value. We would be appalled, Buxton says, if substantial funding were top-sliced from monies allocated for direct patient care to promote the rapid dissemination through the NHS or a novel, largely unproven diagnostic technique. The introduction of medical audit can, however, be likened to such a scenario.

Clinical audit and the 'science cycle'

Bhopal and Thompson (1992) argue that to make audit more effective it should be integrated into the science cycle. This refers to the need to summarise knowledge, formulate standards and methods for audit, to conduct the audit using valid and reliable data collection methods and statistically calculated sample size, to make results available using easily assimilated graphs, conduct workshops to agree changes and then repeat the whole cycle again. Adequate and appropriate support structures are similarly necessary for successful audit (Bhopal & Thompson 1992), and Buxton (1994) is clear in pointing out that the skills necessary to achieve effective audit are not yet readily available in many of the contexts in which routine audit is required.

Identification and characterisation of methodological deficiencies in audit practice

The recently published work of Buttery *et al.* (1994) provides a useful assessment of the current status of audit practice in English provider organisations. The authors report that 79% of provider units responded to their survey, representing 325 provider units out of 411 surveyed. This enables a detailed characterisation of audit progress which extends earlier research conducted by Hopkins (1993; 1994). The following lists qualitatively describe 30 principal deficiencies that are evident from this published research (data derived from Hopkins 1993; 1994; Buttery *et al.* 1994).

Audit committees

(1) Role of chair of committee not analysed and defined.
(2) Lack of involvement of chair of committee in training others in audit.
(3) All committees chaired by medical staff with 'medical domination' of the constitution.

(4)   Size of committee interfering with the decision-making process and optimum size undefined.
(5)   Lack of 'executive clout'.
(6)   Lack of clarity of relationship of committee to provider management and to purchaser.
(7)   Lack of establishment of Nursing and Midwifery and/or clinical audit committees.
(8)   Clinical audit committees created by simple addition of nursing and therapists to existing medical audit committees.
(9)   Under-representation of nurses and therapists on established clinical audit committees.
(10)   Non-representation of patients or their representatives.

Planning

(11)   Proposed audit projects not systematically and critically appraised for relevance and usefulness before resources committed.
(12)   Discussions about whether or not to support specific audit projects made on case by case basis without any properly defined criteria or framework to support decision making.
(13)   Failure to involve chief executive, director of nursing/quality, managers and purchasers in audit planning.
(14)   Planning had little reference to the wider needs of provider organisations; audit committees and specialities determined their own agendas, priorities and objectives.
(15)   Failure to demonstrate forward plans for audit and lack of review of performance against planned objectives.

Method and design

(16)   Most audit projects did not involve collection of large sets of data – sample size of many medical audit projects was typically quite small.
(17)   Case note review, not systematic audit, most frequently employed form of audit.
(18)   Need for further research into audit methodology identified.

Data and IT

(19)   Reliability of data and role of IT uncertain.

Implementation

(20)   Deficiencies in follow-up and implementation of agreed policies.
(21)   Advice relayed to management frequently ignored and lack of shared vision evident.
(22)   Difficulty in persuading management to take action on recommendations made in 'audit reports'.

Relationships to quality assurance and R&D

(23)   Lack of integration of audit with provider quality initiatives, particularly to complaints mechanism and the Patient's Charter. Audit generally not employed to implement evidence-based clinical practice.

Integration with continuing clinical education

(24)   Inadequate links between audit and postgraduate education.

Audit departments

(25)   No consensus on how audit departments should be structured, organised and managed.

Audit staff

(26)   No consensus exists on the necessary skills, background, training and grading of audit co-ordinators and associated staff.

Reporting and accountability

(27)   Written reports of audit activity not available in all cases.
(28)   Reporting to management minimal with 'autonomy' of audit in some cases.
(29)   Reporting to purchasers 'rare'.
(30)   Audit committee chairmen more likely to report good performance to management than bad performance.

The need for a systematic method for critical inquiry into clinical practice

The identification of deficiency is the first stage in its correction. The second stage is the development of methodologies which are designed specifically to preclude identified deficiencies and the logical ordering of those methodologies into a system aimed at guaranteeing the success of healthcare audit, and its functional integration with provider research and development (R&D) and organisational quality assurance (QA) programmes. A detailed characterisation of broad deficiency affords a fundamental opportunity for formulation of 'best', or at least 'better', methodological practice in audit through, in part, detailed reference to the established ineffectiveness of recent and historical approaches.

The model presented here is based on this philosophy. The overall methodology is presented as an algorithm (Figure 3.1). Each guideline is parenthetically numbered and its individual rationale is discussed in sequential fashion accompanied by detailed methodological guidance in each case. The presented method is delineated into the following five components:

- systematic forward planning of audit
- systematic design of audit
- stage 1 audit
- implementation of change
- stage 2 audit.

A detailed illustration of the presented method is given in Figure 3.2. This chapter considers 11 guidelines which specifically consider the managerial structures and organisational innovations necessary to establish audit infrastructure within healthcare provider organisations. Guidelines 11–20, presented in Chapter 4, specifically discuss methodologies for management of process and measurement of outcome.

Guideline 1: Trust board adds chair of clinical audit function to portfolio of medical director

Responsibility for audit

Buttery *et al.* (1994) observed that the role of the chair of the audit committee has never been formally defined or analysed. They noted that, of the total number of audit committees examined, 97% were chaired by medical staff, most of whom were of consultant grade. Of this percentage, 14% were identified as clinical directors and 5% were medical directors of the provider unit. The chair of the clinical audit function carries the ultimate responsibility for the creation, approval and operational implementation of audit policy. The chairman steers audit and is therefore its primary director.

Published research clearly demonstrates that most audit committee chairs have been frustrated by their apparent inability to achieve change through operational means, that is, by their lack of executive authority (Hopkins 1993; 1994). Indeed, Hopkins (1993) observes that 'the leading problem appears to be … lack of executive clout', with advice relayed to management being ignored and accompanied by a lack of shared, corporate vision. Hopkins observes that audit committee chairs felt their committees would benefit from 'more teeth', with the need expressed for stronger links between management and medical staff in the exercise of audit.

Buttery *et al.* (1994) note that audit chairs were more likely to report good performance in audit to management than bad performance. This indicates that the Trust board's lack of direct involvement in the business of the audit committee can lead to inadequate reporting of audit and to what Buttery *et al.* (1994) refer to as 'an unduly rosy view of the development of audit'. Indeed, the same authors demonstrate considerable deficiencies in the nature and extent of reporting audit findings to management, but note that audit is more likely to be discussed at Trust board level if a board member is included in the constitution of the audit committee. Provider organisations with a section on audit in the unit business plan are also more likely to discuss audit at board level and more likely to have a board member on their audit

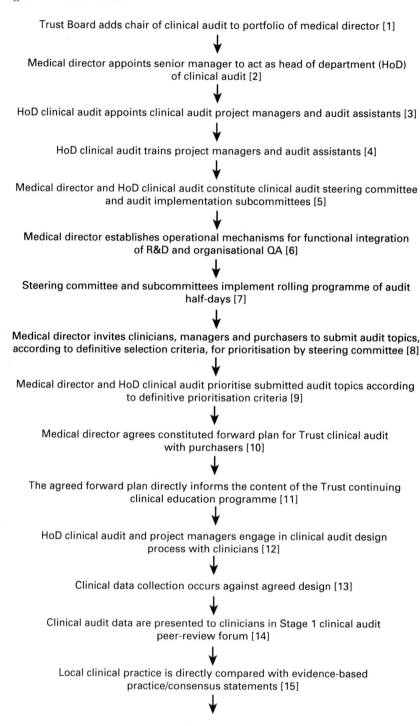

Trust Board adds chair of clinical audit to portfolio of medical director [1]

Medical director appoints senior manager to act as head of department (HoD) of clinical audit [2]

HoD clinical audit appoints clinical audit project managers and audit assistants [3]

HoD clinical audit trains project managers and audit assistants [4]

Medical director and HoD clinical audit constitute clinical audit steering committee and audit implementation subcommittees [5]

Medical director establishes operational mechanisms for functional integration of R&D and organisational QA [6]

Steering committee and subcommittees implement rolling programme of audit half-days [7]

Medical director invites clinicians, managers and purchasers to submit audit topics, according to definitive selection criteria, for prioritisation by steering committee [8]

Medical director and HoD clinical audit prioritise submitted audit topics according to definitive prioritisation criteria [9]

Medical director agrees constituted forward plan for Trust clinical audit with purchasers [10]

The agreed forward plan directly informs the content of the Trust continuing clinical education programme [11]

HoD clinical audit and project managers engage in clinical audit design process with clinicians [12]

Clinical data collection occurs against agreed design [13]

Clinical audit data are presented to clinicians in Stage 1 clinical audit peer-review forum [14]

Local clinical practice is directly compared with evidence-based practice/consensus statements [15]

Fig. 3.1   The 20 stages associated with successful completion of the audit cycle.

Changes in clinical practice are agreed and aimed at reducing the identified discrepancy between local practice and evidence-based practice/consensus statements [16]

Agreed changes in clinical practice are implemented with generation of process outcomes and publication of interim results [17]

Clinical audit data are presented to clinicians in Stage 2 clinical audit peer-review forum [18]

Clinical benefit deriving from implementation of practice change is quantitatively measured and qualitatively described [19]

Outcome measures are published in clinical press and Trust contracting plans [20]

committee. Furthermore, Buttery *et al.* were able to demonstrate a clear association between the type of audit methodology employed and the profile and importance afforded to audit within provider units. For example, those provider units including audit in their corporate business plans, with board representation on the audit committee and showing some sort of strategic organisation of audit (e.g. a forward plan), were less likely to be using mortality/morbidity review and more likely to be using more systematic methods.

Need for a Trust board member on the audit committee

It seems clear, therefore, that the presence of a board member on audit committees begins to address effectively the under-developed links between audit and management. This having been shown, it remains to be established what status the board member should hold on the audit committee, again with direct reference to the concerns that have been articulated and the difficulties that have been reported. If these concerns and difficulties are to be productively addressed, the audit committee chair must develop (or already have) strong links with executive management in order to secure an executive authority not only in theory (which would be of little use in a function so operational as audit), but also in practice. The strongest links with the Trust board are, of course, *integral* links. The medical director of the Trust has such integral links and is a functioning interface between management and clinicians who can therefore preserve clinical leadership of audit.

Arguments against the exercise of audit chairmanship by the medical director

Some investigators including Miles *et al.* (1996b) have argued against the role of audit chair being taken by the medical director of the Trust on the basis that the medical director is unlikely to hold the position of

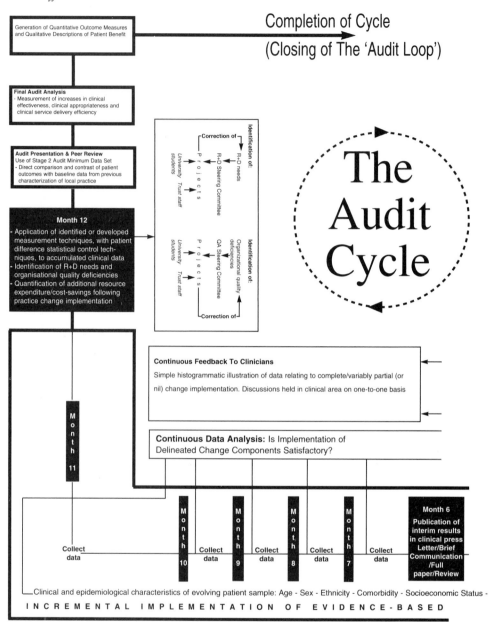

Fig. 3.2 Diagrammatic illustration of the audit cycle, modelled according to the methodology described.

postgraduate tutor and that a firm link with postgraduate education is necessary. It has been argued that the committee chair should be a distinguished academic, for example a professor of medicine or surgery, so that the philosophical link of audit and continuing clinical education can be duly symbolised. The medical director is part of management and some clinicians argue that audit is not. Too promi-

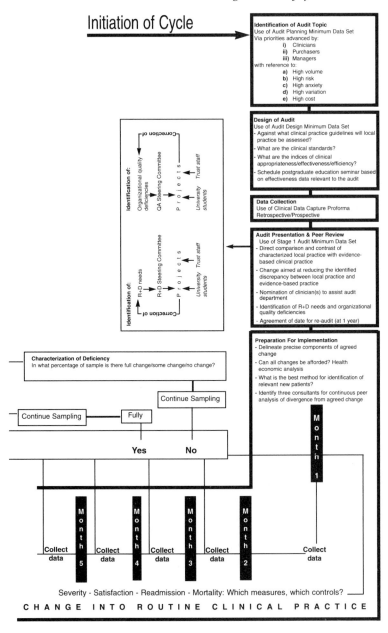

nent a role of management in audit is 'dangerous' because it remains unclear to what use management will put audit findings. The medical director would also be able to 'style' audit according to the requirements of management and not to the requirements of the profession locally.

A key philosophy in this argument is that the medical director has a substantial interest in maintaining the acceptability of clinical services within the provider organisation and in increasing their quality. The medical director may therefore be biased towards favouring the selection and performance of audits which 'show the quality of service in a good light', while systematically deselecting audit topics that aim to address areas of poor clinical quality. The contention is, therefore, that medical directors would selectively and particularly employ audit to demonstrate their own effectiveness, and this may be detrimental to the core function and development of audit. A combination of the roles of audit committee chair and medical director would, they say, pre-dispose to a direct conflict of interest.

'Styling' of audit by the medical director

The objection that a medical director will 'style' audit according to the requirements of management should not, however, afford concern. Provider management is concerned with the continuing viability of the organisation from which comes the employment of all staff, including the clinicians'. It is axiomatic, therefore, that any management requests made to the medical director in terms of priority areas for audit are likely to be directly concerned with this viability and as such should automatically be supported by the clinical staff. Even in these cir-cumstances, the medical director's responsibility for audit can com-plement more general responsibilities. The medical director is the most managerially prominent clinician and would therefore be able to argue on an even footing against an audit that has been suggested by the Trust board but which may be considered unnecessary or unethical by clinicians. Such opportunities would not normally be available to any other clinician exercising the chairmanship of audit. Indeed, in these circumstances, that clinician might simply receive an instruction from the Trust board and not have easy access to the executive forum in which to argue against it.

It should be remembered that the medical director has only one loyalty, a loyalty that acts to guarantee his colleagues' future by doing his part to secure the continued viability of the provider organisation. He is unlikely to compromise himself or his colleagues using the audit mechanism. The objection that he will employ the audit mechanism to show the clinical service in a 'good light' may appear to be sustainable on the basis that the medical director is substantially concerned with the viability of the organisation and this will depend on the quality of its services, which index directly affects the maintenance of existing contracts and the winning of new ones. However, audit is by its nature conducted using data generated by clinicians who are aware of the general characteristics of those data and exercise a relatively high level of so-called data ownership in this context. It is extremely difficult for the medical director to be able to manipulate audit findings in any way without precipitating scandal amongst his colleagues. Even if the medical director were prepared to divest himself of all professional and moral integrity he would still find himself rapidly exposed by any attempt to manipulate a process which is so substantially owned by the clinical staff. Indeed, short of being powerfully and universally charismatic, he would experience considerable difficulty in securing a co-operation of clinical colleagues so great as to allow an ongoing, corporate deselection of negative audit findings.

The medical director is empowered to act executively in the operational implementation of audit policies. The medical director is able to allocate resources accordingly and is also well-placed to overcome the pockets of consultant resistance that are a well-recognised feature of audit implementation and development. He is able to effect changes in the established patterns of clinical activity to ensure that adequate time is made available for audit and is able to counsel consultant medical staff who consistently do not fulfil their contractual obligation to participate in audit.

The medical director is therefore able, in direct fashion, to address the frustrations expressed by clinicians that:

- management does not act on, and effectively ignores, audit findings
- management does not allocate the necessary resources to implement findings
- management holds little interest in audit.

The primary ability to empower and implement changes indicated necessary by audit may be considered by some to be considerably more valuable, at least initially, than a primary ability to link audit with continuing clinical education. Indeed, the latter can be achieved through other mechanisms which are described subsequently in this text and it is a prominent responsibility of the postgraduate tutor to ensure that this happens. In most provider organisations the postgraduate tutor is, anyway, responsible to the medical director for the exercise of that function.

On the basis of this reasoning and with reference to the findings of research (Hopkins 1993; 1994; Buttery *et al.* 1994) it is concluded that the role of chairperson of Trust audit is best exercised by the medical director, to which role it is highly complementary. With reference to research and to the increasingly recognised requirements of the clinical audit process, six principal functions of the audit committee chairman become evident and these are advanced as the suggested basis of a typical description of duties.

(1) The motivation and education of all clinical staff in the meaning and purpose of audit.

(2) The creation of a culture change where audit is recognised as an integral, not additional component of good professional practice.

(3) Steering of clinicians away from the view that case review and the medical round are acceptable forms of audit and towards the recognition of audit as formally described by the Royal Colleges and Department of Health.

(4) The planning of audit with direct reference to the priorities of

clinicians, management and purchasers, which priorities should be essentially similar.

(5) The operational implementation of changes in clinical practice, evidence-based where possible, with the allocation of the resources necessary to effect that implementation.

(6) The securing of outcomes from audit which show, in a tangible manner, that increases in the quality of care have occurred, of direct benefit to patients within the provider organisation.

Guideline 2: Medical director appoints senior manager to act as head of department of clinical audit

Adequate support is an essential prerequisite in securing the success of operational audit. This is typically provided by audit support staff, working collectively in an audit department. To conduct audit with acceptable frequency in all medical specialties and in all healthcare professions operating within the provider organisation, a significant level of intellectual, organisational and clerical support is required. Without clerical resource, clinical data of statistically acceptable volume are unlikely to be collected by busy clinicians. The clerical support is likely to be provided by basic grade administrative and clerical staff, typically NHS Administration and Clerical Grade 3 (A&C 3), and with reference to their functions the title audit assistant(s) is recommended.

Without some form of organisational management, this clerical support will be unco-ordinated on a day-to-day basis and integrity of data will be unassured. Management of the clerical resource and a form of overall co-ordination of operational audit is therefore required and this can be exercised by middle-grade administrative and clerical staff (A&C 5/6) who, with reference to their functions, are best described as project manager(s). Without a definitive intellectual input, the project managers (and certainly less so the audit assistants) are unlikely to have a clear idea of what clinical data to collect, how data should be aggregated, how they might be interpreted in consultation with clinical staff and, importantly, how scientific papers are written for publication in the clinical press. In addition to operational audit, there will be a need to implement, maintain and develop a functional integration of clinical audit, R&D and organisational quality assurance programmes, and a need to link audit with continuing clinical education.

The individual required to exercise these functions will need to have very particular skills. These will range from the ability to ensure the generation of quantitative measures of improved patient outcomes across all clinical services on the one hand, to basic staff management on the other. Also vital is the ability of this individual to gain the confidence of senior clinical staff and the Trust board through personal credibility and subsequent achievement. As a consequence, this person is likely to be selected from candidates with a higher degree, preferably a doctorate, in an appropriate scientific discipline, such as medical laboratory sciences, medical informatics or a clinical discipline involving a high level of knowledge of medical science and statistics. The demonstration of a high order of communication skills, both verbal and in writing, is to be considered essential.

The performance objectives of this position will mirror those of the medical director for audit implementation, maintenance and development and a description of duties for recruitment purposes can be constructed easily from this text. The individual will therefore be directly accountable to the medical director. Direct accountability is highly desirable, not only from the point of view of enabling the medical director legitimately to give instructions and to set tasks, but also because it demonstrates that the individual is 'clinical property' and not an element of what might otherwise be viewed by clinicians as an inappropriate managerial structure within the clinical audit process.

The necessity for this post derives from the recognition that it is impossible for the medical director to exercise day-to-day management of what is essentially a large, complex function of the Trust requiring full-time commitment, reading and research. With reference to these complex operational and developmental functions and to the likely seniority required to attract an individual with corresponding abilities, it is recommended that this function is best described under the title Head of Department of Clinical Audit with SMP grading likely to be made within the range SMP 14–19, depending on local circumstances.

Guideline 3: Head of department of clinical audit appoints project managers for medicine, nursing & midwifery and therapies and clinical support services, plus clinical audit assistants: constitution of a Trust department of clinical audit

Staffing of clinical audit departments

No consensus exists on the necessary skills, background, training, entitling and grading of audit co-ordinators and associated staff. There is also a similar lack of consensus on how audit departments should be structured, organised and managed (Buttery *et al.* 1994). The staffing of provider medical audit departments and its associated training issues has been examined by Buttery *et al.* with the observation that human resource represented the largest single cost of audit programmes in 1992/1993, consuming 39.1% of available audit monies.

Audit staff are employed for three principal reasons:

(1) They are recognised as possessing some skills necessary for audit that clinical staff do not possess.
(2) They can function as data collection and input staff, functions which would otherwise be an uneconomical and inappropriate use of clinical time.
(3) They can function in the general management of the audit

programme and in the dissemination of information, organisation and provision of training and in the collation of reports on audit activity (Buttery *et al.* 1994).

Organisation of appointed audit staff: provider departments of clinical audit

Buttery *et al.* (1994) observed that in 75% of audit programmes, audit personnel were managed within a central audit department from which services were provided to the organisation as a whole. Departments were typically managed by an audit co-ordinator who was a member of audit staff with varying managerial responsibilities for the audit department and for the audit programme in general (although in some circumstances audit departments were directly managed by the chairman of the audit committee or by another member of unit senior staff such as the Director of Nursing/Quality). The authors observed that in 16% of audit programmes, some audit staff, although centrally organised, were separately managed within individual departments, directorates and specialties. The balance of centrally placed and out-posted audit staff showed considerable variation between provider units. Buttery *et al.* observed that in 9% of audit programmes, no central department existed and audit staff were completely devolved to specialties or departments. It is advanced here that audit departments should be centrally administered under the management of the head of clinical audit. This will ensure standardisation of approach and consistency of progress and is considered vital to the systematic development of clinical audit within provider organisations.

Guideline 4: Head of department of clinical audit trains project managers and audit assistants

Clerks, administrators and senior managers who are of necessity involved in the audit process must be adequately trained if success is to be achieved. Currently, the greatest percentage of audit clerks, officers and facilitators come from inadequate backgrounds and are of insufficient grade (Miles *et al.* 1996a, b). This directly affects their ability to undertake key functions associated with the audit process, which range from the simple to the very complex (Kent 1994; Buttery *et al.* 1994; Miles *et al.* 1996a, b). Clinical audit staff are often dedicated and hard-working, but effort and ability are easily distinguished. The demand for training from these individuals and the continued variability in the criteria for appointment selection are noteworthy observations in this regard. Barnes *et al.* (1994) are clear in stating that

'most healthcare professionals have never had any proper training in quality improvement and audit. The limited training available has often been focused on a single technique (such as standard setting). It has rarely given participants a structured overview of the quality improvement process and provided them with all the skills they need'.

The need for careful, explicit training is thus axiomatic.

Guideline 5: Medical director and head of department of clinical audit constitute clinical audit steering committee and audit implementation subcommittees for medical audit, nursing & midwifery audit and therapies & clinical support services

Clinical audit steering committee

Buttery *et al.* (1994) observed that less than a third (29%) of audit programmes were directed by a clinical audit committee. Many (31%) had some form of combination of medical and other audit committees, and 39% had a medical audit committee only. The authors report that the membership of all types of audit committee demonstrated a very high level of representation from medical staff, particularly from acute specialties, and virtually all audit committees were chaired by a doctor of consultant status – a finding in agreement with Hopkins (1993; 1994). Specifically, Buttery *et al.* report that almost every respondent (98%) confirmed the existence of an audit committee as part of their audit programme and, in some cases, diversification of membership into the non-medical healthcare professions was observed.

Constitution of audit committees – general observations
Buttery *et al.* (1994) speculate that the constitution of audit committees within provider units affords a useful index of the progress made towards implementation of multidisciplinary, that is, clinical audit. Indeed, these authors point out that, in the 39% of programmes where only a medical audit committee existed, it was unlikely that adequate support structures and systems aimed at developing audit in the nursing and therapy professions were present. The authors felt that the existence of a nursing and therapy committee in addition to, but quite separate from, the medical audit committee, might represent a useful index of the extent to which audit was being developed in the nursing and therapy professions, but also an index of the minimum extent to which cross-profession, multidisciplinary audit collaboration was occurring.

Buttery *et al.* (1994) observe that all of the committees responsible for medical audit programmes – irrespective of whether or not they were meant to be clinical audit committees – demonstrated a high level of representation from medical staff, a finding in agreement with Hopkins (1993; 1994). Indeed, Buttery *et al.* report that 75% of the membership of medical audit committees and 53% of the membership of clinical audit committees were medical staff, with the remaining membership of audit committees consisting of audit staff (9%), managers (7%), nurses (5%) and other clinical professionals (5%).

Buttery *et al.* also examined other potential categories of membership that were unrepresented. They found that 65% of committees did not include representation from junior medical staff, 61% did not include representation from the therapy professions and 51% did not include representation from the nursing profession. Only 2% of all committees surveyed failed to include representation from consultant medical staff (Buttery *et al.* 1994).

Sizes of audit committees

Examination of the relative sizes of medical audit committees and clinical audit committees within provider institutions has revealed interesting results (Buttery *et al.* 1994). Clinical audit committees were generally of larger size than medical audit committees, with a mean of 19.0 members versus 15.5 members, respectively. Many clinical audit committees appeared to have been created by the simple addition of a limited number of representatives from the nursing and therapy professions, and on this basis the authors were unsure of the ability of such clinical audit committees to pursue and manage a truly multi-disciplinary audit programme.

Solid infrastructure is a fundamental prerequisite for proper implementation, maintenance and development of clinical audit within provider organisations. A central committee structure through which policy can be translated into practice is therefore essential in the organisation of the clinical audit function. A committee structure is recommended which is nuclear in size, representative of all healthcare professions operating within the provider organisation and which is directly associated with the Trust board through the firm leadership of the Trust's medical director. The steering committee should be small enough to ensure efficient decision making, while at the same time large enough to ensure the representation of the non-medical professions and other agencies.

The recommended constitution of the clinical audit steering committee is shown in Figure 3.3. The pivotal importance of the chairmanship of the committee by the Trust's medical director has already been fully discussed (Guideline 1). The rationale underlying the appointment of the remaining members of the committee is presented below following a description of the nature and function of the audit implementation subcommittees.

Membership of the clinical audit steering committee

Audit implementation subcommittees

The audit implementation subcommittees are so named to describe their nature and function in representing:

- organs with responsibility for recommending policy to the steering committee and for implementing agreed policy changes in clinical practice

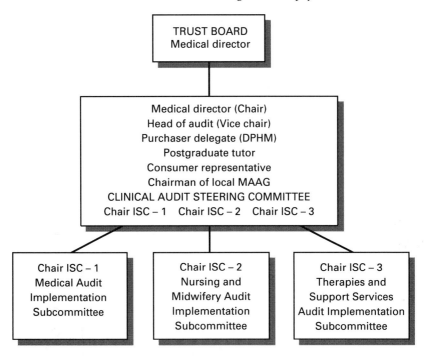

Fig. 3.3 The organisational relationship between the Trust board, clinical audit steering committee and the audit implementation subcommittees.

- legitimate professional concerns in relation to audit implementation and development.

The chairs of the audit implementation subcommittees have automatic membership of the steering committee. This ensures a direct line of communication between clinicians and the chair of the steering committee and hence to the Trust board by virtue of the regular role of the steering committee chairman as medical director. Such automatic membership also creates the core multidisciplinary nature of the constitution of the steering committee. In this way, the dual need to keep the committee small enough to manage, but big enough to be fully multidisciplinary, is satisfied. The multidisciplinary constitution is, moreover, a highly functional one and is therefore essentially different from the typical audit committee constitutions in many English Trusts. These have elected for the cosmetic addition of nurses, allied professionals and managers onto an existing medical audit committee, subsequently referring to the altered structure as a clinical audit committee, but in real terms creating only a medical audit committee 'in disguise'.

The constitution and terms of reference of the audit implementation subcommittees are shown in Table 3.1, using the medical audit implementation subcommittee as an example. The principles of constitution and terms of reference are cross-applicable to the other subcommittees described.

Table 3.1 Constitution and terms of reference of the medical audit implementation subcommittee.

Constitution

(A) Consultant representatives for major medical specialties operating within the Trust.
(B) Head of department of clinical audit.

Terms of reference

(1) To meet at the beginning of each operational quarter and to submit a quarterly report with recommendations to the clinical audit steering committee.
(2) To ensure active participation of all doctors in medical and clinical audit through monitoring of attendance levels and exertion of peer pressure.
(3) To maintain compliance with the Trust audit strategy in consultation with the clinical audit steering committee and department of clinical audit through exertion of peer pressure.
(4) To monitor the extent of implementation of agreed changes in clinical practice in consultation with the clinical audit steering committee and department of clinical audit.
(5) To consider the significance to patients of process and final healthcare outcomes deriving from implementation of agreed changes in clinical practice.

Chairmen of the audit implementation committees (AICs)
There must be separate chairmen for each subcommittee, that is the medical audit implementation subcommittee, the nursing & midwifery audit implementation subcommittee and the therapies & clinical support services audit implementation subcommittee.

The data generated through the functioning of the audit process are very considerable, in terms of actual volume, as well as clinical and scientific complexity. These data cannot be considered in their entirety by the audit steering committee or by the medical director outside of the committee forum, and support structures which are operational rather than strategic in nature are therefore necessary. Meeting at the beginning of each operational quarter, the audit implementation sub-committees have responsibility for professional audit within their own remit, thus protecting professional concerns and helping to minimise professional anxieties in relation to rapidly evolving multidisciplinary audit. The chairmen of these subcommittees have automatic right of membership of the steering committee which meets at the end of each operational quarter and is therefore able to receive the business of the individual subcommittees. The steering committee is therefore truly multidisciplinary in constitution and represents an ideal forum for agreement and planning of professional audit.

Audit plans and policies, agreed in the steering committee, can be taken back to individual professions by the individual subcommittee chairmen, and strategic agreement can be translated into operational action. The description of the subcommittees as 'implementation sub-committees' is therefore useful in reflecting both their function and accountability. Figure 3.3 has illustrated the extent to which communication between the Trust board, steering committee and audit implementation subcommittees is streamlined by the constitution described.

Chairman of the local medical audit advisory group (MAAG)

The quality of clinical practice, although tightly associated with the delivery of care, and therefore with *process*, is nevertheless intimately associated with *clinical outcome*. The immediate effects of acute clinical intervention in the hospital setting are representative of only one element of the patient experience and it is clear that adequate examination of the long-term outcome of clinical intervention is of central relevance when auditing the quality of the totality of patient care.

Communication between the secondary and primary healthcare settings is recognised as being inefficiently organised. Such inefficiency negates attempts to facilitate continuity of care, interfering with the ability to maximise the benefits of acute care and often precluding the ability to characterise long-term clinical outcome. Representation of the primary healthcare setting at the level of the steering committee is highly desirable therefore and, from the particular perspective of audit, is best exercised by the chairman of local GP audit, that is, the chairman of the medical audit advisory group (MAAG). The involvement of the MAAG chairman in the work of the steering committee acts to link audit planning, design and execution in the community, with audit being planned, designed and executed in the hospital. It facilitates the discussion of the appropriateness and scientific adequacy of audit within each setting and directly enables local GP concerns to be represented to the hospital. Furthermore, it enables local GP concerns to be translated into audit projects within the hospital through joint planning, and facilitates the scale and extent of audit through pooling of joint resources for given audit projects. Audit of the primary–secondary interface is made a possibility through such a mechanism.

Postgraduate tutor

Hopkins (1993) has investigated the relationship between audit and postgraduate medical education, observing the clinical tutor to be in many cases a member of provider audit committees and in a few cases its chair. It appeared from this research that the tightness of the link between audit and postgraduate education depended simply upon the particular degree of interest in audit held by a given postgraduate tutor. If the tutor were interested in audit the link might be strong, but if he were not the link might be weak. The research showed that some institutions attempted to establish a link by holding audit meetings in postgraduate medical centres, but this might represent only a geographical and symbolic link rather than anything particularly functional and may therefore be of no real intrinsic value. Hopkins (1993) reports the comments of one audit chairman that 'audit projects are not of sufficient impact to ensure much of a stir in postgraduate education.' That a great deal of audit so far conducted has lacked this weight may be one reason underlying inadequate integration to date.

The authority to practise comes from society, and both the public and politicians require clinicians to perform competently. Hayes (1995) is clear that to perform satisfactorily a professional needs to be competent, but reminds us that many things can come between that competence and the performance of the clinician. These will include resources such as time, staff and facilities, the functioning of the clinical team as a whole and possible behavioural factors. Hayes is similarly clear in stating that performance can be measured by medical and clinical audit and that this provides a better basis for assessing individual and team requirements for continuing education than that provided by central committees. Hayes has pointed out that adults learn best when they recognise they have a need to learn, following recognition of the relevance to learn in a given area. Hayes argues that continuing medical education is best designed in response to the findings of local medical and clinical audit. It effectively ensures that clinicians do not restrict their continuing education only to topics that interest them, instead establishing a complementarity between their education and the needs of the clinical organisation.

Kerrison *et al.* (1994), in an examination of the relationship between audit and continuing clinical education in provider organisations, observed that the link between audit and postgraduate education did not warrant the description 'tight' or 'functional'. Hayes (1995) emphasises that clinical audit represents a valuable opportunity for reassuring the public about medical performance and to provide an indication of medical education needs. Hayes is clear in stating:

> 'Linking audit and peer review to continuing medical education would allow anxieties about the effectiveness of continuing medical education to be addressed, would permit local ownership, and would allow doctors to choose learning methods that meet their educational needs and fit in with their personal learning styles. Such a link would avoid the need to introduce sanctions because with audit as the monitoring instrument, participation and the attainment of satisfactory standards of performance would be documented'.

Hayes (1995) recognises that the identification of learning needs through audit findings is 'ideal', though such idealism can only be translated into reality if adequate methodological measures are taken to ensure a functional link of audit with continuing clinical education. The presence of the postgraduate tutor on the steering committee is the first step in creating such a functional integration. Using such attendance and the discussion possible through it, it is possible to forward-plan monthly seminars focusing on clinical effectiveness and evidence-based clinical practice as part of the established continuing medical education programme. Topics for the sessions are derived from the topics within the Trust audit programme. Seminars may be delivered on, for example, the role of thrombolysis in acute myocardial infarction, steroids in pre-term labour, and thromboprophylaxis in orthopaedic surgery. The sessions should be delivered jointly by a consultant in the given specialty who concentrates on the purely clinical aspects of the presentation and by the head of department of clinical audit who concentrates on the scientific nature of the findings, for example the scientific integrity of the data forming the medical effectiveness literature and the processes of derivation of evidence such as formal meta-analysis (Guideline 11).

Director of public health medicine (DPHM)

In their examination of the status of audit progress in English providers, Buttery *et al.* (1994) demonstrate an essentially minor involvement of purchasers of healthcare services in the planning and management of clinical audit in English provider organisations. Chapter 8 of this volume considers the role of the purchaser in particular detail and the reader is referred to it for a comprehensive discussion. It is advanced here that the purchase of healthcare should be followed automatically by audit of product. Purchasers are now beginning to respond to this philosophy in that a great many are actively concerned to ensure that their providers are including areas of established clinical effectiveness in the audit agenda.

It is further argued here that the agreement of the content of the audit agenda should form an integral part of the clinical audit contract between providers and their purchasers, and in the handing over of monies for clinical audit. Clearly, purchasers should have an appropriate forum in which to communicate these and related concerns. It is logical, therefore, for the local director of public health medicine to be afforded full membership of the steering committee. In this way purchasers are able to inform the audit agenda with epidemiologically indicated local (as well as national) health needs, and they also have a continuous overview of the progress of audits which they have requested. In this way, they can assist in the interpretation of the results. After all, public health physicians are trained in techniques that are proving increasingly important in the audit process. If research needs and organisational quality needs are indicated by such audits (see Guideline 6), they may similarly be discussed with the purchaser in this forum.

Purchased healthcare: contracting and monitoring through commissioned audit

Rumsey *et al.* (1994) emphasise that the processes of contracting for clinical audit and for monitoring of clinical audit are inextricably linked. They are clear that a contract for clinical audit between the purchaser and provider is probably of little practical use if it is devoid of effective and appropriate monitoring mechanisms. These investigators have recently characterised the nature and extent of purchaser involvement in provider clinical audit in 86 of 123 purchasing authorities identified in England. They report that in 83% of the purchasing authorities examined, the monitoring of audit was undertaken by the Department of Public Health Medicine. In the greatest majority of purchasers, this department was additionally responsible for negotiating the clinical audit contract, mainly (thought not exclusively) in discussions between the director of public health medicine and the chair of the provider medical audit committee (63%).

Rumsey *et al.* (1994) report that the monitoring of clinical audit by purchasers was largely 'reactive and paper-based' and relied rather heavily on receipt of written reports. Commissioners confirmed that they received some form of progress report in relation to provider audit, but the quality and completeness of the supplied information was generally held to be unsatisfactory and approximately half of responding purchasers felt the reports they received had failed to identify any real quality improvements resulting from audit. Rumsey *et al.* observe that commissioners generally received retrospective information pertaining to audit (for example, annual reports), rather than prospective information (for example, forward plans). As the authors point out, this may be an important limiting factor on the ability of commissioners to influence the direction and management of audit programmes.

Indeed, Rumsey *et al.* observe most commissioners to be dissatisfied with the standard of the monitoring information they received from provider organisations. Commissioners are reported to have expressed a strong interest in receiving better and higher quality information in relation to provider audit. They were particularly concerned to receive information relating to the audit process itself and of the changes and improvements in the clinical service resulting from audit. As a member of the steering committee, the director of public health medicine is able to participate in the forward planning of audit, introduce topics of particular concern, and receive and discuss data on audit in process.

Purchasing of management packages: role of commissioned audit and the director of public health medicine
Charlton (1993) has predicted that the targets and priorities in *Health of the Nation* and *First Steps for the NHS*, both published in 1992, will inevitably be incorporated into purchaser–provider contracts and that 'the next logical step will presumably be to enforce these protocols at the level of individual practice'. As a consequence, Charlton argues, clinical decision making which has been autonomous, will have to occur with direct reference to management, possibly through direct accountability. In more specific terms, this translation of priorities into contracts will involve NHS purchasers contracting with NHS provider units for highly specific clinical management packages.

Charlton (1993) points out that one of the principal functions of district health authorities and family health services authorities will therefore be 'to manage the translation of scientifically established knowledge into NHS practice', despite the profound difficulties inherent in any simplistic approach that the exercise of this function may involve. Charlton envisages a situation where the identification of a significant medical advance by purchasers or by the NHS Management Executive will lead to an automatic introduction of change into routine practice. This might be achieved through insistence by purchasers on the development of local protocols which, when developed, can be further modified to ensure uniform best practice.

Charlton views this predicted scenario as a managerial device for successful implementation of 'top down' change. Although the process is promoted as making medical practice more scientific, Charlton believes that at its basis lies a significant conceptual error: it is simply not how science works. The core nature of the concern articulated by Charlton is based on the need properly to understand the relevance of clinical guidelines to patient care in the local clinical setting. If purchasers recommend through the contracting process that provider units 'support and stimulate the development of guidelines and policies' for the thrombolytic treatment of acute myocardial infarction, few, says Charlton, would disagree with the wisdom of this therapeutic principle. However, on face-to-face contact with the clinician, some patients will not prove suitable for simple pre-existing algorithmic treatment. In these cases the necessary exercise of clinical judgement will cause a guideline contravention that would be detected automatically by an audit system such as that described here (see Chapter 4, Guideline 17). Is such a contravention valid? Should it be paid for? These are questions which may well arise and which would warrant discussion with an appropriate member of the purchasing team. The director of public health medicine is, axiomatically, the most appropriate agent in this context and his presence on the steering committee is important when discussing, understanding and resolving such disputes.

There is also the problem of guideline validity to be discussed between purchasers and providers as part of audit administration. Hayward (1994) is clear that the use of contracting to change clinical practice would be an entirely unevaluated method and one which has a 'mechanistic' feel. Much has been written in the literature of 'unscientific practices' and 'outdated treatments', but the purchasing of care (perhaps via financial mandate), through guidelines that are premature or controversial or already outdated, is equally unsatisfactory. As Charlton (1993) points out:

> 'real breakthroughs are rare and the temptation will be to overuse the system to enforce politically acceptable, rather than scientifically valid, practices'.

There is a risk within every provider organisation that this will prove to be the case, so the importance of an adequate forum to discuss the adoption or rejection of particular sets of available guidelines is evident. Since the audit mechanism has been more or less clearly identified as an effective means of guideline implementation, especially using the method advanced here, the forum for discussion of these concerns is ideally provided by the clinical audit steering committee. Recommendations made at this level may then proceed to the provider clinical policy committee. The importance of the presence of the director of public health medicine in such a forum is therefore immediately apparent and enables concerns to be directly and frankly discussed.

Consequences of failure to achieve a proper partnership with the director of public health medicine

If mutual understanding is not achieved between providers and purchasers in relation to the most appropriate, efficient and effective means for delivery of healthcare (O'Neill *et al.* 1996), the relationship will become to a greater or lesser extent adversarial (Thomson 1994) with purchasers being viewed by providers as a 'foreign irritant to be neutralised' (Donabedian 1988). This will generate defensiveness and antagonism in provider clinicians (Thomson 1994). The establishment of a proper co-operative relationship and the attenuation or preclusion of 'clinical defensiveness' and 'clinical antagonism' is greatly facilitated by the presence of the director of public health medicine as a full member of the provider clinical audit steering committee. The additional danger in excluding the director of public health medicine from the membership of the steering committee may be a reciprocally 'aggressive' and 'antagonistic' position of the purchaser as a consequence of being starved of everything but minimal morbidity and mortality data (Wareham 1994a, b). This would be an unsatisfactory situation and would be attenuated or precluded by adequate communication with an appropriate member of the purchasing team. This is clearly the director of public health medicine.

Objections to full partnership with the director of public health medicine

Some clinicians will disagree with the extension of full membership of the steering committee to the director of public health medicine and, as Roche (1994) has said:

> 'would be reluctant to release audit results at the point where a problem has been identified, but would be willing to share the results of the completed projects, after remedial action has been taken and a change in practice demonstrated'.

This is clearly too ideal a situation and the fact that the purchaser will see 'bad' as well as 'good' audit results, may encourage clinicians to implement remedial measures at a more rapid rate than that traditionally associated with operational implementation of practice change. That the purchaser, through the representation of the director of public health medicine, should be afforded this privilege is vital. It is equally vital that purchasers employ sufficient sensitivity in their reaction to such results. In commissioning audits and examining their results, purchasers should ask the question: 'Can this hospital provide good quality care?', and not, in simplistic fashion, 'Does this hospital provide good quality care?' (Wareham 1994a, b).

Any approach by the purchaser that lacked sufficient sensitivity would clearly destroy any feelings of trust and confidence that may have existed to that point. It would have the same effect as would the success of a lawsuit based on negative audit findings: profound medical anxiety, defensiveness and antagonism. In the same way that there should be *ipso factor* granting of public interest immunity in cases of attempted medico–legal use of audit findings, purchasers should also refrain from unduly negative comments or punitive measures following examination of 'bad' results in the forum and papers of the audit steering committee. Indeed, it is well established that co-operation generates better results than coercion or frank conflict (Axelrod 1990). Hayward (1994) believes that:

> 'Purchasers need to have a more interactive role: they need to establish dialogue with local hospital doctors, general practitioners and patients.'

The constitution and function of the clinical audit steering committee, with its representation of a local consumer, the chairman of the local MAAG and the chairs of the audit implementation subcommittees, provide this specific opportunity for the purchaser through functional dialogue with the director of public health medicine in the forum of the clinical audit steering committee.

Consumer representative

Robinson (1994) points out that medical audit has focused over-whelmingly on 'the scientific and technical aspects of quality, rather than on equity or humanity' and quotes the study by Berg and Kelly (1981) which examined 60 000 criteria employed in 448 audits with the demonstration that only 3% related to psychosocial aspects and 4% to communication with patients. Indeed, as Donabedian has pointed out, the interpersonal aspects of healthcare are seldom evaluated, although their importance is unequivocal (Donabedian 1988; Robinson 1994). Rigge (1994) concurs and feels that

> 'too many audits are based on patients as cases, as members of diagnostic related groups, as the subjects of medical records'.

In Chapter 11 of this volume, Rigge asks 'whose outcome is it anyway?' and is concerned that the rhetoric of 'patient empowerment', 'consumer involvement' and 'patient-focused care' is translated into reality (Rigge 1995).

It is fair to say that the issue of consumer involvement in the management of the audit process is a difficult one because most patients have a limited understanding of clinical issues and the traditional means of expressing legitimate concern has been via the formal complaints mechanism. It is, of course, gratifying that as a result of the initiative of investigators such as Rigge, the patient view is no longer considered by doctors as 'inherently fallacious' (Chilton *et al.* 1978). It would certainly be fallacious to state that patient and clinician views of appropriate therapy inevitably coincide (Frankel 1991).

The presence of a consumer representative on the steering committee is highly complementary to the role of the director of public health medicine as purchaser representative. In this way, the purchaser as buyer of healthcare and the patient as consumer of healthcare are both present in the actual setting of healthcare delivery. This might be considered the first stage in establishing a functional involvement of patients in the healthcare audit process. Writing in Chapter 11, Rigge augments her previous thinking (1995) in talking of the relevance and availability of evidence-based medicine to patients.

Guideline 6: Medical director establishes operational mechanisms for functional integration of R&D and organisational quality assurance activities

Studies have demonstrated that a substantial quantity of audit funding has been used by clinicians to undertake clinical research. This has resulted from various factors including a confusion of audit with research (Bhopal & Thomson 1992), and the perception of research but not necessarily audit as a worthwhile and intellectually challenging pursuit (Thomson & Barton 1994).

Clinical audit and clinical research

In discussing the integration of research and audit, it is necessary to understand the quintessential difference between these functions. In understanding their differences one can more readily understand their complementarity, and thereby the philosophical basis for their functional integration in operational practice, a factor advanced as central to the development of quality of clinical care. It is noteworthy that the audit function has frequently been substituted by research and not assisted by it. Clinicians are often reluctant to demarcate these functions despite the clear and fundamental differences that separate them. Research is devoted to the extension of knowledge and audit is devoted to the use of that knowledge in operational practice. The complementarity of the functions is therefore explicit.

Bhopal & Thomson (1992) have elegantly articulated the differences and similarities between audit and research. These authors agree that research and audit are complementary activities and that co-operation between them, rather than competition, is necessary since both are problem-solving activities requiring rigorous methods and reliable, valid data to achieve results. Quintessentially,

'if research is about discovering the right thing to do and audit about whether the right thing is being done and is achieving results, then the interrelationship between audit and research is clear'.

(Bhopal & Thomson 1992).

A synergistic interrelationship between audit and research may be seen to exist between these activities in health services and the creation of a functional relationship between them results in a mutual enhancement of the utility of each.

It has also to be remembered that the interrelationship of audit and research can be converse in that audit, in characterising the deficiencies and variations that occur in clinical practice, can stimulate research (Bhopal & Thomspon 1992). An interrelationship between audit and organisational quality assurance can similarly be described. It may take the form, for example, of the Trust complaints mechanism identifying trends in clinical complaints which can subsequently be utilised in informing the audit forward-planning process, generating priorities for clinical audit. Similarly, audit may identify other problems with quality assurance, such as deficiencies in the integrity of NHS clinical information (for example clinical coding inaccuracies, omissions and irregularities in the medical and clinical records (Heath 1986), unacceptable delays in other clinical (and non-clinical) administrative systems). When these and related deficiencies are identified through the audit mechanism, they can stimulate the formulation of quality deficiency correction projects.

Calman (1992) has pointed out that many participants in audit programmes would not immediately recognise the close relation between their activities and a (general) quality assurance programme. As a consequence, Calman argues,

'there is a risk that several disparate activities can be simultaneously underway, based on quite different concepts of quality, with the potential for conflict and duplication of effort'.

So, as Moss and Garside (1995) have rightly concluded,

'the disadvantage of the divided views and approaches to quality that are endemic within the NHS is that the potential capacity of any group alone to improve quality is limited. Any approach to quality improvement in healthcare, to have any chance of success, has to be integrated'.

Integration of provider quality initiatives with clinical audit

Moss and Garside (1995) have pointed out that in healthcare, 'quality' has traditionally been understood in terms of 'clinical quality', and that an implicit distinction has therefore been made between managerial and clinical activity. These authors are convinced that the separate introduction and development of the various quality initiatives in the NHS has contributed directly to an accentuation of the 'different notions of quality' that follow 'traditional tribal divisions' within hospitals. As prominent examples, the authors cite the rather typical scenario of doctors taking responsibility for audit, nurses taking responsibility for quality assurance programmes (including complaints and Patient's Charter) and managers taking responsibility for clinical risk management.

Buttery *et al.* (1994) have examined the extent of integration of provider quality initiatives in terms of two specific areas of organisational quality assurance activity: the Patient's Charter initiative and the complaints mechanism. The authors were able to document that in 70% of medical audit programmes, projects relating to patients' complaints had never been included and that an important source of data relating to quality of care was therefore remaining unutilised. Projects based on Patient's Charter concerns had not been included in 39% of medical audit programmes. The investigators observed no real difference in the extent of such integration between acute, community/psychiatric and combined audit programmes, but did observe an important difference between audit programmes directed by a clinical audit committee relative to a medical audit committee, with the former demonstrating a greater interest in Patient's Charter and complaints activities than the latter. The authors speculate that the low level of integration might reflect a reluctance of clinicians to foster involvement in what might be held by them to be managerially led quality initiatives or, alternatively, that managers had failed to invite or to secure a high level of clinical involvement in those activities.

Buttery *et al.* are clear that the maintenance of such a division does not benefit the provider institution and, with reference to the differences identified between clinical and medical audit committees in relation to integration, anticipate that the shift to clinical audit within provider units will increasingly address this problem.

It is advanced that Trust clinical audit must interrelate with Trust organisational quality assurance programmes and, vitally, with R&D. Without such integration, there will continue to be unacceptable delays in the implementation of evidence-based medicine into routine clinical practice because the need to implement the research will not be functionally associated with the clinical audit that enables it to take place (Haines & Jones 1994; Moss & Garside 1995). Similarly, data from Patient's Charter monitoring and from the results of clinical complaint investigation, will not be considered fully if the quality assurance function remains uncoupled from the audit process.

Requirement for a mechanism which will integrate audit, quality and research in provider organisations: implementation of research data and QA standards using audit

A mechanism is therefore required through which these three separate processes may be functionally integrated in operational practice. The methodology advanced here is essentially simple. Research implementation processes and quality assurance development processes may both be integrated with the clinical audit function in direct fashion through the audit planning process and their incorporation into the forward-planned audit agenda. In this way, effectiveness data from meta-analysed large scale clinical research (such as thrombolysis, salicylate and beta-blockade usage in acute myocardial infarction) can be introduced into the audit agenda as *Audit of management of acute myocardial infarction.*

Known areas of quality deficiency within the organisation such as those described above can be studied by audit. When audit plans are translated into operational audit following the audit design process, effectiveness research must form the basis of the standards against which local clinical practice will be audited, changes agreed and implemented, and health outcomes subsequently measured. Quality assurance standards, locally set following discussion and agreement with purchasers, can similarly be introduced into operational audit in this way.

Generation of research priorities and QA deficiencies by audit

In the same way that research findings and quality assurance standards can be *fed into* the audit agenda, so they may *come out of* the audit process. Indeed, operational audit can identify priorities for research within the organisation (e.g. *whether* a particular intervention was appropriate in the given clinical circumstances, or *why* something should have been the case, or *what* is required to develop a given system. It can then reveal quality assurance deficiencies which warrant correction (e.g. clinical coding deficiencies, medical record retrieval deficiencies, medical record legibility deficiencies and incompleteness of clinical records in terms of omitted or lost detail).

Simple mechanisms for integration of audit, quality and research in provider institutions

To achieve integration, two 'management instruments' are required to partner the clinical audit steering committee. These 'management instruments' are represented by an R&D steering committee and a quality assurance steering committee. Like the audit steering committee, these committees should be 'think tank' in nature and 'nuclear' in size. Their constitutions should be created by the specific selection of individuals within the Trust who have established reputations for excellence in the areas of expertise important for the exercise of the committee functions.

Cross-communication between the steering committee and an increase in the tightness of integration is ensured by the occupation of vice-chair of each steering committee by the head of department of clinical audit. The chairman of the research committee and the quality committee is recommended to be the medical director of the Trust, further establishing a solid integration of the three functions. In the process, a firm, strategic direction is ensured and, as with clinical audit, a direct link with the Trust board is created with the previously articulated benefits of this direct accountability. Like the clinical audit steering committee, the R&D steering committee and the quality assurance steering committee meet on a quarterly basis. The committee structures are shown in Figure 3.4 and the interrelationship of audit, research and quality assurance is shown conceptually in Figure 3.5.

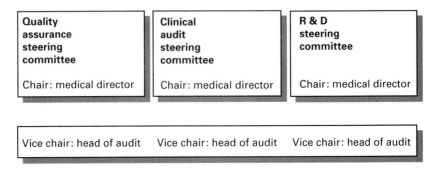

Fig. 3.4 The 'managerial instruments' for functional integration of clinical audit, research & development and quality assurance.

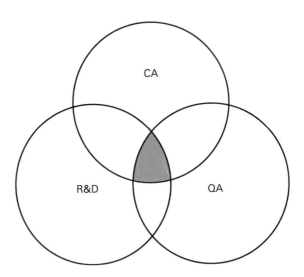

Fig. 3.5 Conceptual diagram illustrating the functional interrelationship of clinical audit (CA), research and development (R&D) and organisational quality assurance (QA) within NHS provider organisations.

The operational mechanism by which such interaction can begin to occur is essentially simple. In addition to the research data and quality standards that can be implemented into routine practice through audit, a mechanism must exist for treatment of the research needs and the quality improvements that are indicated necessary during the audit process. The Stage 1 audit minimum data set (see p. 67) and the Stage 2 audit minimum data set (see p. 67) both ask specific questions in relation to research indications and quality deficiencies: 'What R&D needs have been identified by this audit?' A further question asks: 'What Quality Assurance deficiencies have been identified by this audit?' The indications listed are then directly and automatically transferred to the agendas of the respective R&D steering committee and quality assurance steering committee.

The transfer of these listed indications is then followed by prioritisation and translation into appropriately designed projects. This will involve the QA and R&D committees inviting the Trust quality officer and the Trust R&D officer (or other designated individuals) to formulate draft project designs outside the committee forum in consultation with the department of clinical audit and to submit the drafts for approval and modification at the next respective meetings. If urgency exists, the chairman's action may be obtained from the medical director. Progress reports on a monthly or quarterly basis, depending on project profile and local circumstances, are then made available to individual Trust areas and to the quarterly meetings of the relevant committees. The interim and final results of the projects can then be acted upon by appropriate managers within the organisation, with the advice of the respective steering committees.

Each clinical audit project, when in progress and at the time of completion, can be expected to generate a considerable listing of research and quality improvement priorities, requiring a substantial level of additional resource to enable them to be addressed. Indeed, it is unlikely that sufficient spare capacity will exist in the organisation to undertake such initiatives. How, then, will this extra resourcing be achieved? An appeal to purchasers for specific funding is one option but, routinely, it is recommended that new university links are built or existing ones are extended in order that university students can be allocated to the specific research and quality projects that will be indicated necessary by most audits. An undergraduate student might be allocated to a relatively short-term project of limited complexity while a postgraduate student at the master's or doctorate level might be allocated to longer-term projects of increased or advanced complexity.

University students are a particularly valuable resource in that they represent intellectually able, highly motivated individuals who need to work within the limited, defined timescales of their degrees. University students need data for their theses, experience of the workplace and career references if they are to compete successfully in the marketplace. A typical Trust can offer these benefits in return for the dedication of the student and can also, depending on local arrangements, contribute expenses or offer free or reduced price accommodation to the student in nursing/medical quarters. The university link will also afford the Trust access to specialised facilities and expertise which will range, for example, from statistical support and health economics advice on the

Stage 1 audit minimum data set

(1)   Title (and subtitle, if appropriate) of the audit.

(2)   Name of specialty(ies)/healthcare profession(s)/NHS agencies involved in the audit.

(3)   (a)   Date of meeting.
      (b)   Place of meeting.

(4)   Name(s) of the principal auditor(s):

(5)   (a)   Start time.
      (b)   Finish time.

(6)   Give details of the final methodology employed.

(7)   Give the statistically analysed results of the audit in relation to the indices identified in the audit design minimum data set (Q9–11) for:
      (a)   service delivery efficiency
      (b)   clinical effectiveness
      (c)   clinical appropriateness.

(8)   Give the results from any additional, associated investigations.

(9)   Give results from comparison and contrast of characterised local clinical practice with guideline-indicated clinical practice.

(10) Give details of the local clinical practice guidelines developed as part of the audit (developed *de novo* or developed through local modification of national guidelines).

(11) Give details of the principal points of discussion/contention within the peer-review forum.

(12) Give details of the principal components of agreed change in clinical practice in terms of:
      (a)   clinical service delivery efficiency
      (b)   clinical effectiveness
      (c)   clinical appropriateness

(13) Give details of the methodology to be employed in introducing the agreed changes into routine clinical practice.

(14) Designated clinicians who will work with the department of clinical audit in monitoring and interpreting the extent to which agreed change is being implemented into routine practice.

(15) Nature of anticipated benefit to the patient of implementation into routine practice of agreed changes.

(16) Date set for outcome-evaluating audit (Stage 2 audit) one year after initial practice-evaluating audit (Stage 1 audit).

(17) Clinicians (and others) attending the audit (give names, grades and specialty/profession).

(18) Clinicians not present but scheduled to attend as members of the specialty/profession being audited (give names, grades, specialty/profession and reason for non-attendance).

(19) What were the R&D needs identified by this audit (list in point form)?

(20) What were the organisational quality assurance deficiencies identified by this audit (list in point form)?

Stage 2 audit minimum data set

(1) Title (and subtitle, if appropriate) of the audit.

(2) Name of specialty(ies)/profession(s)/NHS agencies involved in the audit.

(3) (a) Date of meeting.
    (b) Place of meeting.

(4) Name(s) of the principal auditor(s).

(5) (a) Start time.
    (b) Finish time.

(6) Give details of the final methodology employed.

(7) Give details of the statistically anlaysed results in terms of quantitative changes above/below baseline (Stage 1 audit) in:
    (a) clinical service delivery efficiency
    (b) clinical effectiveness
    (c) clinical appropriateness
    that may have occurred as a consequence of the introduction of the agreed changes (Stage 1 audit minimum data set: Q12) into routine clinical practice.

(8) Give a qualitative description of the benefits to patients that have resulted as a direct consequence of the changes detailed in Q7 above.

(9) Describe in quantitative terms the changes in clinical outcome that have been produced locally as a direct consequence of the changes detailed in Q7 above.

(10) Give precise details of the statistical measures employed in controlling for principal inter-patient differences.

(11) Give details of the principal points of discussion/contention as part of the outcome evaluation in the peer-review forum.

(12) Clinicians (and others) attending the audit (give names, grades, specialty/profession).

(13) Clinicians not present but scheduled to attend as members of the specialty/profession being audited (give names, grades, specialty/profession and reason for non-attendance).

(14) What were the R&D needs identified by this audit (list in point form)?

(15) What were the organisational QA deficiencies identified by this audit (list in point form)?

one hand to colour printing and publishing facilities (often of particular use to non-teaching hospitals) on the other. This symbiotic relationship between the NHS and academia is therefore to be highly recommended.

University students are not the Trust's only source of manpower for research and quality projects. Trust staff are increasingly interested in pursuing part-time undergraduate and postgraduate study and it is only reasonable that if Trust staff wish to take advantage of the usual financial contribution and approval of study leave given by the Trust for this purpose, they must select the topic for their undergraduate dissertation/postgraduate thesis from the continually growing list of research and quality projects generated by the audit process. Since audit will be multidisciplinary it is likely that such research and 'quality correction' work will be available within their own area of professional training. If staff decline to focus their studies on an area of identified Trust need, it is recommended that the Trust does not contribute to associated fees. This recommendation might appear somewhat Draconian but in the modern NHS it is important that staff are both patient-focused and organisation-focused. Selection of study areas from a list of Trust research and quality priorities is consistent with this disposition.

This functional interface between clinical audit, R&D and organisational quality assurance is of integral significance in modern methodological approaches to clinical evaluation and is advanced as the platform from which measurable increases in the clinical *effectiveness* and *appropriateness* of care can be delivered *efficiently* to patients. This conclusion concurs with that of Moss and Garside (1995) who are clear that improvements in the overall quality of healthcare are likely to be achieved only through an approach which integrates previously separate 'quality activities'.

Guideline 7: Steering committee with audit implementation subcommittees implement a rolling programme of audit half days

Miles *et al.* (1996a) have argued persuasively that audit is an integral component of good professional practice. This function therefore needs to be exercised in routine manner.

Martin (1992) and Black and Thompson (1993) have demonstrated that 'lack of time' is a frequently cited reason for failure to undertake routine audit, yet as Thomson and Barton (1994) have pointed out, 'lack of time' is not usually perceived by doctors as a barrier to the research in which they engage. The skills are similar (Barton & Thomson 1993) and the time commitment for research is greater (Thomson & Barton 1994). Thomson and Barton (1994) believe that this situation derives from the perception of research as a 'worthwhile and intellectually challenging pursuit' and in the requirement for a research record within the curriculum vitae of doctors progressing towards NHS consultancies.

The forward planning of audit topics and audit meetings appears to play a significant role in increasing the rate of medical attendance (Buttery *et al.* 1994). A forward-planned programme of meetings dedicated to audit is therefore indicated. Thomson and Barton (1994), however, argue against such an arrangement. These authors believe that

> 'the solution is not to identify ringfenced sessions ... in that way audit will continue to be seen as an activity separate from routine clinical practice. Audit needs to be integrated into daily practice.'

While the philosophy forming the basis of the concern expressed by these authors is clear, it is advanced that an abolition of dedicated audit time would be premature and would represent a negative influence in audit development. Indeed, clinicians are increasingly busy, with varying commitments in varying geographical locations in provider units. A mechanism which allocates specific time for specific audit is advanced as essential in guaranteeing the success of audit. Such a mechanism also needs to ensure that dedicated time coincides for each specialty in the provider organisation. In this way, multidisciplinary audit becomes possible. It must, however, be recognised that dedicated audit time recurring on the same day each month can precipitate difficulties for clinicians who hold particular commitments on a given day. As a consequence, a forward-planned programme of dedicated audit time for audit must be a 'rolling programme'.

The chairman of the clinical audit committee has, as medical director, the executive authority to enable the necessary rescheduling of clinics and operating theatre sessions that will be involved in the inception of a forward-planned rolling programme of dedicated audit time. It is recommended that the medical director does so in consultation with the chairmen of the professional audit implementation subcommittees.

Guideline 8: Medical director invites clinicians, purchasers and managers to submit audit topics according to definitive selection criteria for prioritisation by steering committee

Selection of topics for audit

> Buttery *et al.* (1994) were able to observe that 60% of the respondents to their study had employed some form of written guidelines or proposal forms in selecting audit projects for support by audit departments. These authors noted that in general,

> > 'most decisions about whether or not to support specific audit projects were made on a case by case basis, without any properly defined criteria or framework to support decision making'.

It appeared that there was a significant number of audit programmes where proposed audit projects were not systematically and critically appraised for relevance and usefulness before resources were committed.

Forward planning should result in an audit programme that has planned both uniprofessional and multidisciplinary audit priorities in a comprehensive fashion and in a way which has addressed issues of individual and mutual concern to clinicians, managers and purchasers. It is also important that the audit forward-planning process is not so exhaustive as to preclude its completion on time and the existence of spare capacity for topics to be included mid-year as a consequence of priorities that can arise from local incidents or spontaneously identified needs. This, perhaps, requires a certain managerial art, and one which is exercised with reference to principal resources such as clinical audit staff time. The clinical audit planning minimum data set, below, is advanced as a useful tool in securing a forward-planned Trust audit programme.

Audit planning minimum data set

(1)   Name of specialty(ies)/healthcare profession(s)/NHS agency selecting the audit.
(2)   Topic advanced as a priority for audit (give title and subtitle, if appropriate).
(3)   What is the basis on which the topic has been selected – high volume, high variation in clinical practice, high clinical risk, high clinical anxiety, high clinical cost (please state)?
(4)   Do nationally agreed clinical guidelines exist for the management of care within the area for audit selected?
(5)   Will the audit directly compare and contrast characterised local practice with guideline indicated practice?
(6)   If nationally agreed clinical guidelines are unavailable, will local guidelines be developed and, if so, what is the evidence base on which this development will proceed (give details and journal references)?
(7)   What is the anticipated benefit to the patient of this audit?

Agencies in the forward-planning process

It is no longer appropriate or effective to consider forward-planning of Trust audit as the sole responsibility of medical staff and as an 'activity engaged in by consenting adults within the privacy of provider organisation' (Gill 1993). This improved understanding of the function of the clinical audit mechanism has led to the agreement that forward planning of audit should be a multidisciplinary process. It is advanced here that three principal agencies require involvement in the forward-planning process. These are clinicians, local managers and purchasers.

(1) Clinical professionals
   (i)   Medical staff
      (a) consultant medical staff

   (ii) Nursing staff
      (a) clinical nurse specialists
      (b) ward sisters/charge nurses

   (iii) Professions allied to medical staff
      (a) chief physiotherapist
      (b) chief dietician
      (c) chief occupational therapist
      (d) chief speech therapist
      (e) chief pharmacist

(2) Trust managers
   (i)   medical director
   (ii) nursing director
   (iii) clinical directors
   (iv) care group managers/service managers

(3) Purchasers
   (i)   director of public health medicine

Packwood *et al.* (1992) have gone so far as to suggest that contract specification by purchasers should determine the nature of the audit programme, which would certainly represent a major shift away from the principles of professional and provider control that initially shaped its organisation. While this philosophy stands for itself and is to be debated, there are, as Gill (1993) and Miles *et al.* (Chapter 8) warn, attendant risks associated with this approach.

Criteria for rationalisation of topic selection

Several authors have advanced criteria aimed at rationalising the process of topic selection for audit. Selection of topics by clinicians has traditionally been based on areas of personal clinical interest rather than in accordance with the wider needs of the organisation. As the understanding of the nature and purpose of audit has deepened, the legitimate role of managers and purchasers in the audit process has become increasingly recognised. This has directly facilitated a narrowing of the gap between selection of audits based on pure clinical interest on the one hand, and pure managerial interest on the other. The developing role of purchasers, described in outline above, and in detail in Chapter 8, is proving of further utility in increasing the appropriateness of local audit agendas (Thomson & Barton 1994; Buttery *et al.* 1994).

The literature, at the time of writing, is not over-burdened with guidance in this context, though several notable studies may be cited which have aimed at increasing the likelihood of objective appropriateness of audit agendas. Walshe and Tomalin (1993) advance eight selection criteria for local audits where each criterion is scored from 0 (no, not at all) to 5 (yes, definitely). These authors describe their guidelines as serving two purposes:

(1) Helping to improve the quality and effectiveness of the audit projects undertaken locally.
(2) Providing information in relation to the nature of local audit activity itself, thereby accounting for the manner in which audit resources have been used.

Thomson and Barton (1994) are similarly clear in insisting that audit must be integrated into local and national service priorities, noting that the means of setting priorities and selecting topics for audit have been variable from site to site. These observations are confirmed unequivocally by Buttery *et al.* (1994) who noted that

> 'there are still many audit programmes where few audit projects are systematically and critically appraised before resources are committed to undertaking them'.

It is advanced here that systematic forward-planning of provider audit should occur with direct reference to the five principal and definitive criteria advanced by Shaw (1989) of high volume, high clinical anxiety, high clinical variation, high clinical risk and high cost. The basis of this concurrence, and the simple methods by which each can be achieved, is now addressed.

High volume
In any area of performance analysis it is immediately logical to focus primarily on those areas of practice which are performed most frequently. The effectiveness and appropriateness of clinical practice in these areas and the efficiency with which improvements in these indices are delivered to patients should therefore be studied, and frequently encountered conditions should be automatically selected for audit. Clinicians will, of course, be fully aware of the sort of patients they see routinely, but managers and purchasers can obtain a precise indication through activity analysis. The hospital information system is useful to managers in indicating the top ten diagnoses within each medical specialty practised within the Trust. The computer printout thus obtained for each specialty should then be sent both to the clinical director and service director/manager of that specialty. Discussions should be organised between these individuals and the relevant clinicians, and topics for audit selected accordingly.

High clinical anxiety
Selection of audit topics with reference to areas of high clinical activity represents a sound, initial approach to the formulation of an audit agenda that is sensitive to, and focused on, local health need. Consideration of high activity alone is insufficiently lateral and audit

selection must also examine areas of low volume. This might seem paradoxical but complex conditions often present in low numbers and this factor can predispose to limited logistics for the management of such conditions, with an increased potential for clinical error and reduced quality of care. Problems in this context may have been experienced by clinicians where critical incidents or iatrogenic injury have narrowly been avoided. Where clinical anxiety can be seen to exist, it must automatically inform the audit agenda. Clinical anxiety can be identified *directly* by interviewing clinicians formally (a simple questionnaire) or informally (conversation) with direct, sensitively phrased questions. It can be detected *indirectly* by reviewing death and complication data where formal trend analysis – or in many cases simple observation – demonstrates a recurring problem in the management of given conditions. Depending on the volume of such cases, retrospective analysis may need to examine a three to five year time period.

Some 20 years ago, Rutstein (1976) and associates suggested a quintessentially similar approach. These authors avoided direct questioning of clinicians as a method of establishing activities that they might consider appropriate for audit. Instead, they proceeded by identifying outcome perspectives of clinical practices that demonstrated the need for audit, but which might not otherwise have been advanced by clinicians as suitable for audit. Rutstein outlined a process whereby outcomes that were described as 'sentinel health events' were identified as indicators for audit. The process involved producing a listing of unnecessary diseases, disabilities and untimely deaths. An 'event' might be represented, for example, by the death of an asthmatic patient under 50 years of age.

Examples of areas of clinical anxiety to a diabetologist might be represented by unexplained retinopathy or renal impairment in young, apparently well-controlled diabetics. A haematologist may well hold anxieties when confronted with idiosyncratic resistance to normally effective therapy, for example, primary resistance to chemotherapy in Hodgkin's lymphoma. Selection of audit based on clinical anxiety is particularly patient-focused but is also integrally linked to effective clinical risk management (Vincent 1996).

High variation in clinical practice

The degree of variation in clinical practice between clinicians is often 'startling' (Hopkins 1990) and is considered in Chapter 1 of this volume as a primary area for application of the audit function. Variations in clinical outcome that persist following control for population risk and other key epidemiological factors probably represent definitive differences in the technical effectiveness of clinical care. They may involve differences in the *style* or practice, which in some cases may be independent of the objective appropriateness of intervention and which may ignore the availability of data which show the limited effectiveness of one approach over another. The investigation of clinical practice variations between individual consultant firms in a given organisation is both professionally and morally necessary. Indeed, all patients have the same right to 'best' outcome and should therefore enjoy access to 'best' practice, irrespective of individual consultants or individual Trusts. Identified areas of local variations in practice between consultant firms therefore warrant automatic selection for audit.

Areas of practice variation may be identified by simple comparative analysis of inter-consultant firm management of similar patient case mixes. Topic areas are best selected for audit of practice and outcome variation in the following circumstances

(1)   When national clinical guidelines for best practice are available for given conditions within given specialties.
(2)   When trend analysis of patient complaints reveals dissatisfaction with the outcome of care and where this is associated with a given area of practice in a given consultant firm.

Characterisation of local clinical practice for each consultant firm in the identified areas can then be directly compared with clinical practice guidelines and action taken to reduce the discrepancy between the two.

High clinical risk

The methodology for selection of audits on the basis of high clinical risk shares some principles with the method for selection of audits on the basis of high clinical anxiety. Direct inquiry of clinicians can certainly be employed but is less relevant because the medical specialties of high risk are well known (for example, obstetrics) as are the hospital areas of high risk (for example, delivery rooms and operating theatres). Although the examples given are particularly noteworthy in terms of their prominent association with clinical risk, all clinicians and all hospital areas will share a variable but nevertheless significant clinical risk potential. It is therefore important that the audit agenda is informed accordingly. The methodology with which areas for audit may be selected on the basis of high clinical risk should involve:

- identification of critical incidents: actual and narrowly missed
- identification of patients' dissatisfaction with the outcome of their care associated with a given area(s) of practice in a given consultant firm(s) through trend analysis of patient complaints
- identification of high perioperative mortality
- identification of unplanned returns to theatre related to post-operative complications
- identification of non-adherence to clinical practice guidelines.

When actual or potential risk has been grossly identified in this way, it should automatically inform the audit agenda. Audits may then be designed in order fully to characterise the nature of local practice associated with risk, protective measures agreed and implemented, and decreases in the indices described above, subsequently quantitatively measured.

High cost

Medical staff have traditionally held little interest in the cost of the care they provide and have given preferential importance to the delivery of effective care; they are trained to believe that they should provide *ideal* (rather than *reasonable*) care to the people they have identified as needing it (Buchan 1993). Clinical decisions have immediate resource implications and inadequate reference to the cost of care during the clinical decision-making process, can lead *ipso facto* to delays in access to care of waiting patients until budgets are renewed or while excess costs are being negotiated with purchasers.

Selecting audits with reference to cost effectiveness was discussed as early as 1971 by Delbecq and Van de Ven (1971). Essentially, two meetings were scheduled between relevant clinicians. Individual clinicians were required to advance suggestions for audit which were critically appraised and scored for likely cost effectiveness in improving patient care. The process described is valuable in generating a listing of priorities for audit, with subsequent review of the utility of this procedure yielding positive results (Williamson *et al.* 1979).

Many treatments have been shown to be ineffective, yet are retained by some clinicians. Meanwhile, other expensive treatments are sometimes employed in preference to cheaper options which may be equally or more effective (Haines & Jones 1994). Sometimes, a given alternative treatment may be less effective but not radically so, and its use will remain clinically appropriate with the potential for greater patient access created through quantifiable savings. Clinical guidelines are central to audit of areas of high clinical cost. The selection of areas for audit of high clinical cost should involve:

- identification of therapeutic interventions not in accordance with clinical practice guidelines recognised by the relevant Royal College, where peer approval of the non-adherence cannot be gained.
- identification of therapeutic interventions employed by junior staff not subsequently supported by consultant opinion.

When potential cost-ineffective practice has been identified in this manner, it should automatically inform the audit agenda. Audits may then be designed in order fully to characterise the nature of variations in, for example, local prescribing practices (Gosney & Tallis 1984; Freemantle *et al.* 1995) and in the use of given therapeutic interventions. These are then followed by direct comparison of local practice with recognised clinical practice guidelines that have taken account, in their development, of cost effectiveness as well as clinical effectiveness (Drummond 1995). Cost savings that result from implementation of agreed changes in clinical practice can subsequently be quantitatively measured.

Guideline 9: Medical director and head of department of clinical audit prioritise submitted audit topics according to definitive prioritisation criteria

Strategic direction of audit activity

Buttery *et al.* (1994) have provided important data in terms of the strategic direction of audit within provider units. Of their respondents, 87% confirmed the existence of some form of written plan for the audit programme (1993/4) but one in eight organisations (13%) failed to demonstrate the existence of such a document. These authors noted that although audit committee chairs, committee members and audit staff all contributed to the formulation of strategic plans, relatively few chief executives, directors of nursing/quality, managers, or purchasers had significant involvement. As a consequence, audit planning had little reference to the wider needs of the provider organisation and most audit committees allowed specialties to determine their own agendas, priorities and objectives. Buttery *et al.* suggest that the audit planning process in provider units is 'certainly capable of improvement in many audit programmes'. Indeed, 21% of respondents fell into the category of either having no plan at all or having objectives in plans that were never reviewed, 'which means their value was very limited' (Buttery *et al.* 1994).

The process of audit topic generation described in Guideline 8 will result in a multiplicity of audit topics being returned via the audit planning minimum data set (see p. 70), from which a formal Trust audit agenda must be constructed. This will involve a process of prioritisation with specific reference to the available resources needed to undertake selected audits and with reference to the extent of satisfaction of the audit selection criteria (Guideline 8). The prioritisation process will need to consider local epidemiologically determined health needs and national priorities for health, which will have (or should have) been submitted by local purchasers. This same process must also ensure the representation of all medical specialties and, where appropriate, nursing and the professions allied to medicine.

The selected topics are organised into four programmes of audit so that Programme 1 will begin in operational quarter 1, Programme 2 will begin in operational quarter 2, and so on. The constituted audit programme is then agreed by the Trust board and is presented to purchasers as the basis of a contract for clinical audit. When agreement of the Trust board and purchasers is achieved, the programme is circulated to all other relevant staff as considered appropriate by management locally.

Guideline 10: Medical director agrees constituted forward plan for provider audit with purchasers

The pivotal role of NHS purchasers in the development of the audit function has been discussed in previous guidelines in this chapter, notably Guideline 5. A principal function of the purchaser deriving from the philosophies advanced will be to ensure the appropriateness of the audit agenda. Purchasers must be able to satisfy themselves that purchase of service is followed by audit of product, with particular focus on areas of local epidemiologically determined health need and also national priorities for health. The exercise of this function will have, or should have, contributed to the development and prioritisation of the Trust forward plan of audit. In order to ensure that it has, and to confirm the objective appropriateness of the audit agenda, it is recommended that the agreed audit plan is made the central basis of a formal contract for clinical audit through which monies are transferred to the Trust and into which performance measures (such as completion of audits to timescale and validity criteria) are built. The presence of the director of public health medicine as a member of the clinical audit steering committee ensures that progress can be continually measured according to agreed criteria and that any operational or associated difficulties in achieving progress in such a complex function, such as audit, are discussed and understood.

Guideline 11: The agreed forward plan directly influences the content of the Trust continuing clinical education programme

A laboratory scientist would, as an automatic consequence of his particular training, ask the question 'what is the nature of the existing and recently published data relevant to my work, and how can I be assured of the integrity of those data?' Such a question is incontrovertibly valid and directly relevant to the direction the scientist will give to his ongoing work. The clinician should similarly ask such questions in relation to proposed practice changes: 'Where do these standards and guidelines come from? What is the integrity of the data on which they are based? Is there an expert consensus recommending their use?' The answers to these questions are clearly relevant to the clinician's decisions to use or reject the standards/guidelines. A mechanism within NHS Trusts which will routinely provide the answers to these clinical questions does not so far exist, but an initial methodology is presented within this guideline for the first time. The integral link between education and the success of audit becomes immediately clear in this context.

If clinicians' questions are answered to their satisfaction, acceptance of standards/guidelines and implementation of change become possibilities. If such questions are not answered, the likelihood of change implementation is small. The peer-review forum is too advanced a stage in the audit cycle to be adequate and appropriate for this exercise. It is recommended that such questions are addressed in a recognised, pre-existing programme of postgraduate medical education into which effectiveness/audit teaching can be 'slotted in'. It is suggested that a *new* programme of postgraduate lectures dealing specifically with effectiveness research is not likely to be well-attended, other than by those clinicians with a personal interest in this area.

It is recommended that the sessions should therefore take place *in advance* of the Stage 1 audit peer review and their topics should be drawn directly from the established forward-planned audit programme. An increased familiarity with the topic area will be achieved in this way prior to the Stage 1 audit comparison of characterised local practice with evidence-based practice in the peer-review forum. As a consequence, clinicians will be in a far better position to debate the audit findings in an intellectual manner and are far more likely to understand the relevance of the effectiveness data used in the comparison. It is therefore anticipated that they will be more likely to agree changes for implementation into routine clinical practice than if the educational intervention had not been employed.

Conclusion

The introduction of systematic audit within health services began with the promulgation of a definition and the recommendation of the classical model of audit based on 'structure, process, outcome'. Theoretical concepts are of limited use until they are translated into operational products. Sound knowledge, understanding and methodology are fundamental to achieving such products.

The British NHS did not invest in fundamental research into audit that would have generated a recommended, standardised and comprehensive methodology. A series of evaluations, together with anecdotal observation, demonstrated wide-ranging variations and deficiencies in the approach to audit. No author has demonstrated, in unequivocal terms, an ability of audit to precipitate and maintain changes in clinical practice and to produce measurable, clinically-valid benefits for patients, and until effective audit methodologies are employed, this scenario will not change.

This chapter has sought to examine the management structures and organisational innovations that are prerequisite to effective audit structure in healthcare provider units, advancing associated recommendations in the form of 11 guidelines. Chapter 4 examines the implementation of the audit process and considers the basis for measurement of clinical benefit following audit of healthcare services.

References

Axelrod, R. (1990) *The Evolution of Cooperation*, Penguin, Harmondsworth.

Barnes, J., Parsley, K. & Walshe, K. (1994) Star quality. *Health Service Journal*, 3 November, pp. 20–22.

Barton, A.G. & Thomson, R.G. (1993) Is audit bad research? *Audit Trends* 1: 51–3.

Berg, J.K. & Kelly, J.T. (1981) Evaluation of psychosocial health care in quality assurance activities. *Medical Care* 21: 24–9.

Bhopal, R. & Thomson, R. (1992) Medical audit and medical research. *Quality in Health Care* 2: 274–5.

Black, N. & Thompson, E. (1993) Obstacles to medical audit: British doctors speak. *Social Science and Medicine* 36: 849–56.

Buchan, H. (1993) Clinical guidelines: acceptance and promotion. *Quality in Health Care* 2: 213–14.

Buttery, Y., Walshe, K., Coles, J. & Bennett, J. (1994) *Evaluating Medical Audit: The Development of Audit – Findings of a National Survey of Healthcare Provider Units in England.* CASPE R search, London.

Buxton, M.J. (1994) Achievements of audit in the NHS. *Quality in Health Care* 3 (Suppl.): 531–4.

Calman, K. (1992) Quality: a view from the centre. *Quality in health Care* 1 (Suppl.): S28–S33.

Charlton, B.G. (1993) Management of science. *Lancet* 342: 99–100.

Chilton, C.P., Morgan, R.J., Enland, H.R., Paris, A.M. & Blandy, J.P. (1978) A critical evaluation of the results of transurethral resection of the prostate. *British Journal of Urology* 50: 542–6.

Delbecq, A.L. & Van de Ven, A.H. (1971) A group process model for problem identification and program planning. *Journal of Applied Behavioural Science* 7: 466–71.

Donabedian, A. (1988) Quality assessment and assurance: unity of purpose, diversity of means. *Inquiry* 25: 173–92.

Drummond, M. (1995) The role of health economics in clinical evaluation. *Journal of Evaluation in Clinical Practice* 1: 71–5.

Fowkes, F.G.R. (1982) Medical audit cycle: a review of methods and research in clinical practice. *Medical Education* 16: 228–38.

Frankel, S. (1991) The epidemiology of indications. *Journal of Epidemiology and Community Health* 45: 257–9.

Freemantle, N., Henry, D., Maynard, A. & Torrance, G. (1995) Promoting cost-effective prescribing. *British Medical Journal* 310: 955–6.

Gill, M. (1993) Purchasing for quality: still in the starting blocks? *Quality in Health Care* 2: 179–82.

Gosney, M. & Tallis, R. (1984) Prescription of contra-indicated and interacting drugs in elderly patients admitted to hospital. *Lancet* ii: 564–7.

Haines, A. & Jones, R. (1994) Implementing findings of research. *British Medical Journal* 308: 1488–92.

Hayes, T.M. (1995) Continuing medical education: a personal view. *British Medical Journal* 310: 994–6.

Hayward, J. (1994) Purchasing clinical effective care. *British Medical Journal* 309: 823–5.

Heath, D.A. (1986) The appropriate use of diagnostic services (XII). Medical audit in clinical practice and education. *Health Trends* 18: 74–6.

Hopkins, A. (1990) *Measuring the Quality of Medical Care*, Royal College of Physicians, London.

Hopkins, A. (1993) *Analysis of comments made by chairpersons of medical audit committees in Trust hospitals, DMUs and DHAs in England, Wales and Northern Ireland in response to a questionnaire sent out in October 1992*, Royal College of Physicians, London.

Hopkins, A. (1994) How well are audit committees working: In: *Professional and Managerial Aspects of Clinical Audit* (A. Hopkins), Royal College of Physicians, London, pp. 111–20.

Kent, P. (1994) The role and training of audit co-ordinators and audit assistants.

In: *Professional and Managerial Aspects of Clinical Audit* (ed. A. Hopkins), Royal College of Physicians, London, pp. 105–109.

Kerrison, S., Packwood, T. & Buxton, M. (1993) Medical Audit: Taking Stock, Kings Fund Centre, London.

Kerrison, S., Packwood, T. & Buxton, M. (1994) Monitoring medical audit. In: *Evaluating the NHS Reforms* (eds R. Robinson & J. LeGrand), Kings Fund centre, London.

Martin, E. (1992) Audit in general practice. *British Medical Journal* **304**: 643.

Miles, A., Bentley, D.P., Polychronis, A., Price, N. & Grey, J.E. (1996a) Clinical audit in the National Health Service: fact or fiction? *Journal of Evaluation in Clinical Practice* **2**: 29–35.

Miles, A., Bentley, D.P., Price, N., Polychronis, A., Grey, J.E. & Asbridge, J.E. (1996b) The total healthcare audit system – a systematic methodology for auditing the totality of patient care. *Journal of Evaluation in Clinical Practice* **2**: 37–64.

Moss, F. & Garside, P. (1995) The importance of quality: sharing the responsibility for improving patient care. *British Medical Journal* **310**: 996–9.

O'Neill, D., Miles, A. & Polychronis, A. (1996) Central dimensions of clinical practice evaluation: efficiency, appropriateness and effectiveness I. *Journal of Evaluation in Clinical Practice* **2**: 13–27.

Packwood, T., Kerrison, S. & Buxton, M. (1992) The audit process and medical organisation. *Quality in Health Care* **1**: 192–6.

Paxton, R., McKenna, M., Grant, B., Railton, T. & Pagan, W. (1993) Doing the rumba: guidance on making clinical audit work. *Health Service Journal*, 25 November: 30–31.

Rigge, M. (1994) Involving patients in clinical audit. *Quality in Health Care* **3** (Suppl.): S2–S5.

Rigge, M. (1995) Whose outcome is it anyway: In: *Outcomes into Clinical Practice* (ed T. Delamother). BMJ Press, London, pp. 40–48.

Robinson, M.B. (1994) Evaluation of medical audit. *Journal of Epidemiology and Community Health* **48**: 435–40.

Rumsey, M., Walshe, K., Bennett, K. & Coles, J. (1994) *Evaluating Audit: The Role of the Commissioner in Audit.* CASPE Research, London.

Russell, I.T. & Wilson, B.J. (1992) Audit: the third clinical science. *Quality in Health Care* **1**: 51–5.

Rutstein, M. (1976) Outcome perspectives of clinical practice. *Medical Education* **9**: 228–38.

Shaw, C. (1980) Aspects of audit 1. The background. *British Medical Journal* **280**: 1256–60.

Shaw, C. (1989) *Medical Audit – A Hospital Handbook*, King's Fund Centre, KFC 89/11, London.

Thomson, R.G. (1994) The purchaser role in provider quality: lessons from the United States. *Quality in Health Care* **3**: 65–6.

Thomson, R.G. & Barton, A.G. (1994) Is audit running out of steam? *Quality in Health Care* **3**: 225–9.

Vincent, C. (1996) *Clinical Risk Management*, BMJ Press, London.

Walshe, K. & Coles, J. (1993) Medical audit: in need of evaluation. *Quality in Health Care* **2**: 189–90.

Walshe, K. & Coles, J. (1994a) *Evaluating Audit: Developing a Framework*, CASPE Research Reports, London.

Walshe, K. & Coles, J. (1994b) Evaluating audit: a review of initiatives. CASPE research reports, London.

Walshe, K. & Tomalin, D. (1993) Rain check. *Health Service Journal* **29**: 28–9.

Walshe, K., Bennett, J., Buttery, Y., Rumsey, M., Amess, M. & Coles, J. (1994) *Evaluating Audit: Effective Audit?* CASPE Research, London.

Wareham, N.J. (1994a) External monitoring of quality of health care in the United States. *Quality in Health Care* **3**: 97–101.

Wareham, N.J. (1994b) Changing systems of external monitoring of quality in healthcare in the United States. *Quality in Health Care* **3**: 102–106.

Williamson, J.W., Braswell, H.R. & Horn, S.D. (1979) Validity of medical staff judgement in establishing quality assurance priorities. *Medical Care* **17**: 331–7.

4 ◆ Methods for Auditing the Totality of Patient Care II: Implementation of Process and Measurement of Outcome

Andrew Miles, Paul Bentley, Nicholas Price, Andreas Polychronis, Joseph Grey and Jonathan Asbridge

Introduction

The process of audit is multi-faceted and complex. Improperly managed, it is liable to become dysfunctional at any point, as experience accumulated since the introduction of formal audit in 1989 has so clearly demonstrated (Miles *et al.* 1996a, b). When appropriate infrastructure has been implemented in provider organisations and priorities for audit agreed, the audit process itself may begin. This will commence with the design of individual audit projects and will end with the generation of data which may be employed in outcome measurement. Intermediate components of process will be data capture and collection, data analysis and presentation, and the agreement, implementation and monitoring of change. The discussion and recommendations for audit process and outcome within this chapter are presented as nine guidelines, the first numbered as '12' and the last numbered as '20'. This facilitates numerical continuity with the guidelines for audit structure within the preceding chapter.

Guideline 12: Head of department of clinical audit and clinical audit project managers engage in the design of agreed clinical audit projects with clinicians

Necessity for adequate design of audit

Adequate design of audit is dependent on an adequate understanding of what audit is, what it must achieve for patients, and how it can be used in this context. In 1989, the Royal College of Physicians published the prominent work *What, How and Why*, which presented broad guidance on methodology of audit, with accompanying definitions of structure, process and outcome (Royal College of Physicians 1989). The college considered that medical audit was primarily a mechanism for:

- assessing and improving the quality of care
- enhancing medical education by promoting discussion between colleagues about practice

- identifying ways of improving the efficiency of clinical care.

Appropriate and effective design is fundamental in achieving these aims.

If adequate design of an audit is not achieved, its purpose will be unclear and the audit is likely to collapse, either during its operation, or in terms of the validity and therefore utility of its results. Sometimes, authors will be aware of the limitations of their study and will alert (or perhaps, alarm) the reader:

> 'This [audit involves] a retrospective review of the X-rays and clinical notes. It is a study using small numbers of patients and is not intended to be statistically significant.'
>
> (Edwards *et al.* 1992.)

Such 'qualifying' statements are of particular relevance since they act to preclude the use of resulting data in terms of patient management or organisational change. (It is noteworthy, however, that the study we quote was reported as having changed fracture management.) Where inadequacies of design are less readily detectable (except to the trained, statistical mind), invalid conclusions may be drawn, patient management altered and recommendations made to Trust boards for organisational change. The inherent dangers of inadequate design in clinical audit are thus clear and emphasise the need for rigorous design, requiring a level of statistical and methodological expertise that cannot necessarily be assumed to be automatically possessed by clinical staff, especially in non-teaching hospitals. These facts demonstrate the need for 'academic modulation' of provider audit. This will sometimes be simple and sometimes complex, depending on the given audit, and it indicates the need for a reservoir of appropriate skills in provider audit departments or through established university links (see Guidelines 2–4, Chapter 3). Thomson and Barton (1994) are in agreement on this point, emphasising that the development of skills in audit design is a 'vital investment' before a functional partnership between audit staff and clinicians can be achieved.

Current status of audit design adequacy in provider organisations

Although there has been no detailed study to date of the audit design processes adopted by provider audits, major conceptual and statistical inadequacy is likely to be present. The support for this assumption is derived from observations by Buttery *et al.* (1994) and by Buxton (1994) in terms of the following:

(1) Limited audit sample sizes (and the immediate concern in relation to representativeness and therefore statistical validity).
(2) The lack of standard setting with reference to evidence-based clinical guidelines/expert consensus.
(3) Failure to consider patients as populations and therefore the introduction of intrinsic obstacles to the ability to demonstrate

significant change over time and to an understanding of the effects of care on population.

(4) Failure to sample retrospectively over an adequate time period and to consider seasonal variations in patient presentation.

(5) Failure to apply appropriate exclusion criteria.

Common methods of designed audit: predominance of case review

Buttery *et al.* (1994) have investigated the general methodological approach to audit in English provider units, with interesting results. The authors studied the six most common methods of audit in order to examine the frequency with which particular approaches had been employed during a one-year period of study. They were particularly concerned to study the methods most likely to be employed, those most readily understood and those which were likely to contain both traditional and modern, explicit and implicit, approaches.

Examination of accumulated data demonstrated case note review to be the most frequently employed form of audit in provider units. Buttery *et al.* report that 73% of respondents ranked this activity as '1' or '2' with the next most commonly utilised form of audit employing the criterion-based approach, with 58% of respondents ranking this as '1' or '2'. Outcome measurement was much less frequently employed as was a formal analysis of the incidence of adverse events. Patient surveys represented the least popular of approaches to audit. The authors were able to conclude, therefore, that case note review and mortality/ morbidity review tend to dominate the approaches to audit in provider units.

Sample sizes employed in audit design

Importantly, Buttery *et al.* examined the sample sizes typically employed as part of the audit process in provider units. The authors asked respondents to indicate the approximate size of samples typically employed in their audit over the period of study with interesting results. The authors were able to observe that

> 'most audit projects did not involve the collection of very large sets of data – the sample size of many medical audit projects was typically quite small'.

Strikingly, the authors observed that 56% of medical audit projects undertaken during the year of study had employed sample sizes of less than 70.

Assurance of validity of audit design

The adequate design of provider audit can be assured and developed through use of the audit design minimum data set, listed below. This design tool has the function of stimulating (and sometimes *precipitating*), ideas from clinicians, managers and purchasers in relation to the dimensions of clinical *effectiveness*, clinical *appropriateness* and clinical *efficiency* which constitute the principal elements of quality in clinical practice (O'Neill *et al.* 1996) and which will therefore need to be examined critically by the audit.

Audit design minimum data set

(1) Name of specialty(ies)/healthcare professions to be involved in the audit.

(2) Date set for evaluation of local clinical practice (stage 1 audit).

(3) Title of audit.

(4) Diagnostic/clinical category(ies) to be examined (give ICD-10/OPCS code(s)).

(5) Selection criteria (e.g. age, sex).

(6) Exclusion criteria.

(7) Extent of retrospective (or prospective, if applicable) data collection (e.g. 3/6/9/12 months).

(8a) Total average yearly throughput of patients (identify any seasonal variations in clinical presentation).

(8b) Percentage sample to be taken.

(9) Are there nationally agreed clinical guidelines relating to the areas of clinical care to be audited (give associated journal reference/other source)?

(10) How will characterised local practice be directly compared and contrasted with the practice advanced by the guideline (give details)?

(11) If nationally agreed guidelines are unavailable and local guidelines are to be developed following characterisation of local practice, what is the evidence base on which such development will proceed (give full details and journal references)?

(12) What indices of clinical service delivery efficiency may be audited (please list in point form)?

(13) What indices of clinical effectiveness may be audited (please list in point form)?

(14) What indices of clinical appropriateness may be audited (please list in point form)?

(15) What are the individual data items that will be required to measure within the indices listed in 12–14 above (please list in point form)?

(16) Are additional, associated data required other than those necessary to measure within the specific indices listed in 9–11 above (please list in point form)?

(17) What is the source of the data (e.g. medical records, nursing records, theatre registers, PAS, MIS etc)?

(18) What statistical treatment of the data is anticipated?

Identification of data items for measurement within identified indices of clinical quality

When clinical effectiveness, clinical appropriateness and clinical service delivery efficiency have been considered, and indices with which to measure them developed, the data items required to 'feed' the indices, that is, to enable measurement within them, need to be identified. This is a relatively simple exercise. For example, if one index of clinical efficiency has been advanced as *Interval between arrival in A&E and initiation of thrombolysis*, then the data items required to measure within this index will be (1) clock time (00hr 00min) of arrival and (2) clock time (00hr 00min) of initiation of thrombolysis; the so-called 'door to needle' time. A recognised standard of care can be attached to the interval, for example 25 minutes, in the context of this example. If standards for best practice are not available nationally, practice standards may in the interim be formulated locally and attached to the various indices in the same way. This is one example of an index of clinical service delivery efficiency, but the principle of data item identification for index measurement remains the same if other indices of clinical service delivery efficiency are to be considered, for example:

- interval between arrival and triage
- interval between arrival and A&E medical assessment
- interval between medical assessment and transfer to ward
- interval between transfer to ward and first cardiological assessment

The same principles are applicable to identification of data item requirements for measurement within indices of clinical effectiveness and clinical appropriateness.

Additional data item requirements

In addition to indices of clinical performance such as intervals and their means, medians and ranges, it is also necessary for the design process to consider associated information requirements such as percentages, actual numbers of cases (n), and also 'answers' to given questions such as: 'Does a protocol exist for fast-track admission of patient with suspected MI with the ambulance service and GPs?' or 'Was thrombolysis stopped? If so, why?'

Adequacy of clinical information

It is recommended that all audits should examine the adequacy of clinical documentation, not only for purely clinical reasons which are of central concern, but also for medico-legal purposes. Attention should always be given during the design phase to the potential for developing a minimum clinical information data set. In ensuring completeness of clinical assessment they are of major diagnostic and prognostic importance and play a central role in providing data which can be employed in monitoring the extent to which practice changes are being implemented. Moreover, they represent the first essential step in computerisation of the medical record, which has a range of associated benefits to the hospital clinician. It facilitates ease of reference to existing information during the current patient episode and also on possible re-presentation. It also has benefits for the GP, because a computerised record can be discharged on disc along with the patient and can therefore prove of use in continuing care in the primary healthcare setting. It has additional benefits to clinicians in other hospitals in which the patient might present where a fax of the record from the record-holding clinical organisation could be requested and transmitted, thereby enabling a much more rapid access to appropriate care.

Role of definitions of minimum clinical data

The design process itself should be careful to establish what exactly constitutes minimum clinical documentation data in the routine or emergency assessment of a patient within the area of examination by the audit. If such consideration does not take place, specific questions in relation to whether or not a specific sign or symptom was recorded (perhaps regarded by a given college as *essential* data), cannot be asked during the data collection phase. It is axiomatic that if relevant questions fail to be asked, the answers to them will not be available for the subsequent audit presentation within the peer-review forum. If a clinician should ask in that forum: 'The Royal College of Physicians says that locus of stroke should always be recorded. Are we doing it, and if so, to what extent, and how was its documentation related to prognosis and appropriateness of PAMS referral?', to respond by saying 'We don't know', would hardly be considered satisfactory.

Two approaches may be taken in this context. The first is to ask clinicians directly in the design phase what exactly they would clerk in terms of history in the presenting patient. These specific information items may then be searched for during the data collection phase. So, if a clinician says in the pre-audit design meeting, 'I think locus should always be recorded as part of the investigation and management of acute stroke', the data capturing pro forma will include a question asking the data extractor: 'Was locus recorded?': Yes __No __; if 'Yes', Where ___?

Role of clinical guidelines in establishing minimum clinical data

The second approach involves the use of clinical guidelines. Where clinical guidelines have been developed which specifically detail minimum clinical data, these data should be employed in producing a draft series of *documentation adequacy indices* to which provider clinicians can add clinical data requirements (with reference to the characteristics of local clinical epidemiology, for example, ethnicity or social status) but not remove data that are considered minimum by the guidelines. In the unfortunate instance of patient litigation, the benefits to the clinician and Trust of a patient assessment according to Royal College criteria or local consultant consensus, need no description here.

Where clinical guidelines do not exist, the audit department will need to construct a minimum clinical data set by direct interview with relevant clinicians and by possible additional reference to the most recent medical textbooks and journal publications within the area of interest. Local consultant consensus is a prerequisite for validity of such a data set. In summary, audit of clinical documentation adequacy should involve direct comparison of local documentation adequacy in terms of what is recorded as having been done and what is *not* recorded as having been done, with direct reference to Royal College guidelines, or in their absence to local consultant consensus-based guidelines. Local deficiencies which have been characterised in this way may be minimised, and that minimisation can be quantitatively measured through local agreements to observe the requirements of the data set and through continuing examination of completed minimum clinical data sets over subsequent months (Guideline 17). The clinical standard for documentation should be 100% for all documentation indices recommended by Royal College guidelines or local consultant consensus-based guidelines as 'minimum'.

Operational organisation of the audit design process

In operational practice, the audit design process will begin with the drafting of the design data set in the matter outlined, followed by a meeting with key clinical staff. The meeting is limited to one hour (this might be a lunchtime with basic refreshment provided) where the draft design is examined critically by clinical staff. The process is typically one of 'brainstorming' with the first half of such meetings generally functioning as a period of assimilation of the draft details by clinicians, while the second half is given over to variable levels of debate. Proceedings culminate into a design which can be described as *penultimate* because it will invariably need to incorporate the additions, deletions and modifications that have been advanced during the design session. These should be introduced immediately by the department of clinical audit.

This approach affords the necessary level of involvement of clinicians in audit design, ensures that clinicians take due account of clinical evidence in the design process, and is highly protective of clinical time. The protection of clinical time is of particular importance, given that a major concern of clinicians centres on the amount of clinical time that audit has the capacity to consume (Black & Thompson 1993; Hopkins 1993; Buttery *et al.* 1994). When the design process is judged to have been successfully completed, data capture, extraction and aggregation can commence.

Guideline 13: Clinical data collection occurs against agreed design

The data collection process: clinical data capture, extraction and aggregation for analysis: source of clinical data for audit

Buttery *et al.* (1994) examined the sources of clinical data employed for audit within provider units. They observed that the most frequently utilised source of clinical data for audit was patient case notes, ranked '1' or '2' by 94% of respondents, with the second most frequently used data source being represented by hospital computer systems such as PAS, Casemix or MIS systems.

Capture of clinical data

The clinical data that will be captured, extracted and analysed will be precisely those indicated by the completed audit design minimum data set. The data item requirements detailed on the audit design minimum data set (see Guideline 12, p. 85) are transferred to the data capture pro forma. This process has been described in outline above and is carried out by a clinical audit projects manager. An example of an audit data capture pro forma is shown in Figures 4.1 and 4.2, with the principles involved with delineation of data item requirement for clinical index measurement having been considered above (Guideline 12).

Following agreement of design, and while the audit data capture pro forma is being drawn up, the clinical audit project manager(s) requests a computer printout from the hospital information system. This is designed to identify all patients coded as having been admitted in accordance with the given ICD code(s), over the time period specified

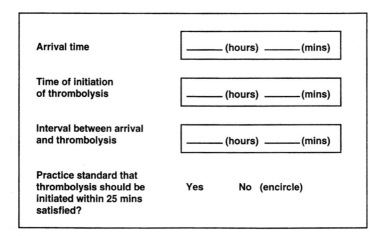

Fig. 4.1 Audit data capture pro forma enabling 'simple level' monitoring of clinical care focused on the so-called 'door to needle' time in acute myocardial infarction.

Time of arrival	_____ (hours) _____ (mins)
Time of establishment of ECG monitoring	_____ (hours) _____ (mins)
Interval between arrival and time of establishment of ECG monitoring	_____ (hours) _____ (mins)
Practice standard for establishment of ECG within 5 mins satisfied?	Yes No (encircle)
Time of completion of twelve lead ECG	_____ (hours) _____ (mins)
Interval between arrival and time of completion of twelve lead ECG	_____ (hours) _____ (mins)
Practice standard for twelve lead ECG to be taken within 15 mins satisfied?	Yes No (encircle)
Time of establishment of IV access	_____ (hours) _____ (mins)
Interval between arrival and time of establishment of IV access	_____ (hours) _____ (mins)
Practice standard that IV access should be secured within 15 mins satisfied?	Yes No (encircle)
Time of commencement of pain relief	_____ (hours) _____ (mins)
Interval between arrival and commencement of pain relief	_____ (hours) _____ (mins)
Practice standard that pain relief should be given within 15 mins satisfied?	Yes No (encircle)
Decision for initiation of thrombolysis recorded in the clinical notes?	Yes No (encircle)
Practice standard that decision for initiation of thrombolysis should be recorded in the clinical notes satisfied?	Yes No (encircle)
Time of initiation of thrombolysis	_____ (hours) _____ (mins)
Interval between arrival and initiation of thrombolysis	_____ (hours) _____ (mins)
Practice standard that thrombolytic therapy should be initiated within 30 mins satisfied?	Yes No (encircle)

Fig. 4.2   Audit data capture pro forma enabling 'intermediate level' monitoring of clinical care focused on the standards for management of acute myocardial infarction in the A&E/Reception phase (Crump 1994).

in the audit design minimum data set. Depending on the method of sampling (sequential, or more usually, random) the project manager uses a highlighting pen to indicate which medical records are to be retrieved. The marked computer printout and also the audit data capture pro forma are then passed to the clinical audit assistant(s) who retrieves the notes and proceeds with the extraction of the data indicated on the drawn audit data capture pro forma.

Briefing of clinical audit assistants immediately prior to the data capture exercise

Prior to actual commencement of data extraction by the clinical audit assistant, the project manager will discuss with the audit assistant the specific clinical terminologies, symbols and annotations that are likely to be encountered to enable recognition and understanding. A system of quality assurance in data extraction is necessary and this takes the form of the project manager independently completing the data capture pro forma for one in five records following their completion by the audit assistant. Direct comparison of the project manager-completed pro forma with the audit assistant-completed pro forma enables a direct data discrepancy analysis and represents a powerful means of identifying any data inaccuracies or data omissions, so that the nature of any errors made by the audit assistant can be characterised and rectified through further briefing.

Clinical input to the data capture exercise

In some circumstances the data extraction exercise will require a definitive clinical input, particularly in situations where interpretation, as opposed to simple observation, is necessary. In such cases, project management will have to ensure that appropriate criteria for interpretation and conclusion are being utilised by the clinician. These criteria should have been considered and agreed by consultant consensus during the design phase. Reproducibility of observation (as a means of data integrity quality assurance) may be tested by ensuring that the participating clinician repeats the interpretations and conclusion that he has already performed and produced, but where he is blind to this exercise. The occurrence of reproduced error due to subjective observer bias may be tested by asking a separate clinician, possibly of consultant status in the same field of expertise, to examine the repeated interpretations, firstly having undertaken the interpretation of that case himself using the objective criteria agreed during the design phase. This exercise is potentially complex (Yerushalmy 1969; Dunn 1989; Sprent 1993; Hripcsak *et al.* 1995) but necessary in circumstances where interpretation is critical to the analysis.

Completion of data capture

> When data collection is complete (within the agreed project management timescale), data are analysed and aggregated in a manner which will satisfy the information requirements of the audit design minimum data set. This may require specialist statistical input in consultation with relevant clinicians, depending on the complexity of the audit. The draft analysis is discussed with the head of department of clinical audit and data are illustrated on OHP acetates or slides in preparation for Stage 1 audit peer review (Guideline 14).

Guideline 14: Clinical audit data are presented to clinicians in Stage 1 clinical audit peer-review forum

Critical analysis of clinical practice: the peer-review process and the consideration of change

> The early models of medical audit emphasised the need for anonymity in audit of medical care and clinical intervention. To maintain confidentiality, NHS management was actively excluded from audit activities and the peer-review forum was created and preserved. Initial guidance on establishing an appropriate forum for confidential discussion of audit findings was described by the Royal College of Physicians (1989).

Criticisms of the peer-review forum

> Some American clinicians and academics believed the process of peer review to be too subjective (Lembcke, 1967; Sanzaro 1974), though the Royal Colleges have adopted and recommended the process as a forum in which full, frank debate can take place. The advent of evidence-based clinical guidelines and a direct comparison of local practice with guideline-directed practice in the peer-review forum addresses the concern of subjectivity. Robinson (1994) points out that the effectiveness of the peer-review process has not been demonstrated by randomised trials, but it is unequivocal that the peer-review process has provided an arena for clinicians to consider each other's practice in a largely constructive, anonymised manner. This has surely been a major advance from the former position of the self-auditing, autonomous doctor, examining his own personal clinical practice in highly subjective fashion.

Clinical perception of the peer-review forum

> It would be untrue to say that the peer-review forum is a universally popular entity; indeed attendance rates are variable both within, and between, provider units (Buttery *et al.* 1994). This may result from the peer-review process being perceived as boring and repetitive (Heath 1990; Gabbay & Laytonj 1992), representing simply a process that

diverts time and energies away from routine clinical practice and the commitment to direct patient care (Robinson 1994). The focus of audit in the early post-White Paper audit definition period was frequently far from what many clinicians would have considered interesting and relevant. Whether the peer-review forum will remain the best method for agreeing changes in clinical practice, or whether one-to-one discussions and 'academic detailing' (Haines & Jones 1994) will prove more effective, remains to be determined. Systematic approaches are currently being undertaken to establish 'best practice' in this context and the results of such research will be highly relevant to progress in the field.

Constitution of the peer-review forum: involvement of the non-medical healthcare professions

Following the establishment of the peer-review forum, the involvement of nursing and the allied professionals became increasingly sought, but represented a source of concern. The importance of nursing and the allied professions in the audit process is growing as a direct consequence of the recognition that audit should embrace the totality of care. In retrospect it seems extraordinary that Halliday (1992) advanced the view that medical audit should be

'an activity carried out by doctors with no input to the process from other groups such as Management or other healthcare professionals, apart from the provision of information'.

As a consequence, audit has moved from self-audit, to peer-review audit, to multidisciplinary audit of the totality of care delivered during the patient episode as a whole.

Need for multidisciplinary involvement in audit and the peer-review forum

Berwick (1989) has reminded us that doctors are not personally involved in the totality of patient care, and Burke (1994) feels that, while the doctor probably knows *more*, he does not necessarily know *best*. Berwick's observation is persuasive and conclusive, emphasising in singular fashion the necessity for multidisciplinary clinical audit. Some anxieties have been largely theoretical. For example, Hopkins (R.) (Ross 1992) has articulated concern in relation to the discussion of surgeons' operation leak rates in a wider forum than a purely medical one. Hopkins' anxiety was addressed by a nurse who had been quoted in conference proceedings as providing the following clarificatory comments:

'who do you think you are kidding? – if you want to know which surgeon is best, or who has the lowest leak rate, ask the nurse because they know perfectly well.'

(reported in Ross 1992.)

Indeed, Ross believes that the idea of four surgeons locking themselves in a room to discuss their results and thinking that other people do not know what is happening, is to be living in 'cloud-cuckoo land'.

Parillo (1995) has provided an interesting perspective on multi-disciplinary care in his presidential address at the 24th Educational and Scientific Symposium of the Society of Critical Care Medicine. He describes in unequivocal terms the importance of a multidisciplinary approach to the care of critically ill and informed patients, emphasising the relationship between best clinical outcome and the multi-disciplinary working of doctors, nurses and allied health professionals. Parillo advances that a qualified critical care physician, possessing the appropriate knowledge, skill, judgement, attitude and compassion acquired through training, experience and a focus on his field should be physically available for patient care without competing obligations. The physician-directed team should manage the environment of critical care, says Parillo, including the 'physical plant', equipment, supplies, personnel and organisation. He is also clear that this multi-disciplinary team approach is not intended to disrupt the relationship between the attending physician and the patient, but that an appro-priately organised (multidisciplinary) intensive care service supports an attending physician in providing the best possible care.

If more than one discipline contributes to care, as is virtually invariably the case in the secondary healthcare setting, then it is insufficiently lateral to antagonise the development of multi-disciplinary audit and therefore the inclusion of the relevant non-medical staff in the peer-review forum. In some areas of care, the separation of the purely medical perspective from the multi-disciplinary aspect of care would represent a clear failure to recognise that

> 'so many interventions depend for their effectiveness on the activ-ities of a team – for example, rehabilitation after stroke. The division between medical and clinical audit [in this circumstance] is artificial and unhelpful'.

> (Royal College of Physicians 1993.)

Nurses and therapists are currently invited to attend typical medical audit meetings in the belief that the presence of non-medical staff, of itself, makes the meeting 'clinical'. In such circumstances the quintes-sential nature of the medical peer-review meeting precludes any meaningful contribution from these groups. Miles (1995a) believes that the development of the *clinical* audit function will depend on critical inquiry into nurses' and allied professionals' practice. 'What, precisely, constitutes best nursing practice in, for example, acute stroke?' he asks. 'What is the minimum nursing data that nurses should record against such practice?' When such questions have been authoritatively and satisfactorily answered, meaningful clinical audit can be conducted, results produced and useful discourse promoted in a multidisciplinary peer-review forum.

Functions of the peer-review forum

It is advanced that the key functions of the peer-review forum are as follows:

(1) To consider characterisations by audit of local clinical practice.
(2) To debate changes in practice based on the various grades of available clinical evidence/expert consensus opinion.
(3) To consider the degree of justification for divergence from agreed changes in practice *during* the change implementation phase.
(4) To consider the nature of clinical change, in quantitative and qualitative terms, *following* implementation of practice changes.

The peer-review forum therefore represents a highly appropriate setting for consideration and agreement of evidence-based practice change. Experience demonstrates that, while setting a date for the peer-review session and securing the attendance of medical staff is all very well, the meeting will need a chair who is able to operate in a specific manner. The chair of the peer-review session is required:

(1) To introduce the meeting and to emphasise the importance of the audit.
(2) To stimulate and maintain relevant discussion of key points.
(3) To steer the peers to agreement on the precise nature and extent of change that is judged necessary, based on the identified discrepancies between local practice and evidence-based practice.
(4) To explain how the agreed changes in clinical practice will be implemented and monitored by the department of clinical audit and relevant peers.

Guideline 15: Local clinical practice is directly compared with evidence-based standards/guidelines/consensus statements

Informal versus formal audit

Many clinicians argue that audit is well-established in clinical practice, citing case reviews and conferences, traditional death and complication meetings and clinico-pathological presentations as evidence in this context. These activities are a form of audit but are to be considered *informal* audit (McColl 1979). In contrast, *formal* audit must involve a detailed examination of clinical practice in a structured, systematic manner with an element of judgement provided normally by one's peers, as well as the previously recognised element of observation. It is at this point in the audit cycle that clinical standards, guidelines and consensus statements are of central significance. The relevance of the recommended design process (Guideline 12) is explicit in this context in that it will have enabled the audit to have been structured in a manner that will allow direct comparison of current practice with evidence-based practice.

What is a clinical standard?

Irvine and Donaldson (1994) have defined clinical standards as complex aggregations of criteria built up into a series of statements describing good clinical practice'. Fowkes (1982) described clinical standards as derivable from clinical experience, textbooks and scientific papers, acknowledging the central importance of clinician participation in standard setting and suggesting a functional role for the Royal Colleges, university departments and 'other learned bodies' in the development of clinical standards.

There is now widespread agreement that clinical standards should be based on clinical research evidence (Haines & Jones 1994; Grimshaw *et al.* 1995). Some clinicians who have, as Rigge (1995a, b) has said 'excessive regard for the sanctity of clinical freedom', remain unconvinced of the merit of this approach and actively debate the concept of individual clinical judgement versus the clinical practice guideline and the applicability of general research evidence to the individual patient. Such issues will continue to attract widespread concern (Charlton 1993; Grahame-Smith 1995; Tanenbaum 1995; Polychronis *et al.* 1996a, b; Klein 1996). Haines & Jones (1994) argue definitively, however, that delays in the implementation of research evidence into routine clinical practice result in suboptimal care for patients, though a conflict need not necessarily exist. In a related context, Godwin (1995) has pointed out that the advance of medical practice will depend on the union of clinical art with high technology science. If practice guidelines are developed with only limited reference to published research, their credibility is limited in parallel and the potential for inappropriate changes in clinical practice is increased. Audit should therefore be centred on evidence-based standards and guidelines (Thomson & Barton 1994; Grimshaw *et al.* 1995).

Relationship of the nature of clinical standards to implementation and use

Fowkes (1982) pointed out that the type of standard developed and selected would represent an important factor in the success of audit. The temptation is to decide on a standard that is optimal, but the ideal is, of course, frequently unrealistic. The example is given of a female patient presenting with symptoms of urinary tract infection. Ideally, one would prescribe an antibiotic based on the result of urinary culture and antibiotic sensitivity testing, though in practice the delay in treatment initiation would frequently be viewed as unacceptable. The *ideal* standard of, say:

'antibiotic therapy in women presenting with symptoms of urinary tract infection will be based on urine culture and laboratory antibiotic sensitivity testing in 100% of cases'

may therefore need to be modified in accordance with practical necessity to:

'antibiotic therapy in women presenting with symptoms of urinary tract infection will have initiated antibiotic therapy maintained or modified with reference to the results of urinary culture and laboratory antibiotic sensitivity testing'.

If such an approach is not taken, an unacceptably low level of adherence to standards is likely to result. This has been recognised for some time. For example, Brook and Appel (1973), in an examination of adherence to clinical standards set by medical academics for the ideal management of urinary tract infection, essential hypertension and peptic ulcer, observed only a 2% adherence. This led Fowkes (1982) to emphasise that clinical standards should be 'realistic and practical for the given clinical situation'.

Minimal versus optimal standards

Having taken account of this factor, Sanzaro (1974) described the use of *minimal* rather than *optimal* clinical standards. Minimal standards are described as being constituted by essential criteria which are represented by 'those elements of diagnosis and treatment which are essential to the proper care of every patient with a specific condition'. It is interesting to see how this early definition has led, through time, to the modern definition of clinical standards as 'complex aggregations of criteria built up into a series of statements describing good clinical practice' (Irvine & Donalson 1994), and the modern definition of clinical guidelines as

'systematically developed statements to assist practitioner and patient decisions about appropriate healthcare for specific clinical circumstances.

(Institute of Medicine 1992.)

Categories of essential criteria

Sanzaro (1974) described three principal categories of 'essential criteria'

(1) Laboratory investigations/clinical documentation of history and physical examination which are of importance in confirming diagnosis, appropriate management and establishing prognosis.
(2) Treatments which are known to be effective.
(3) Treatments (and procedures) known to be contra-indicated.

Again, it is interesting to observe how each one of these criteria has informed subsequent thinking. The first criterion of Sanzaro has led to so-called note audits, perhaps more technically termed *audit of clinical documentation adequacy*, with particular reference (ideally, direct reference) to the minimum clinical data recommended by the Royal Colleges or expert consensus as important for diagnosis, management and prognosis. The importance of such data completeness and integrity in the patient care process is increasingly recognised (Wyatt 1994a–c) and has been recently articulated in an elegant article by Wyatt (1995). The second essential criterion advanced by Sanzaro is now considered incontrovertibly central to good patient care, while Sanzaro's third essential criterion underlies the rapidly developing dimension of clinical appropriateness. It also informs the increasingly important clinical risk management function.

The concept of the 'norm'

Shortly following the consideration of minimal versus optimal clinical standards by Sanzaro (1974), Mintz et al. (1978) advanced the concept of the 'norm', which was a term employed to describe the level of average practice. The essential utility attributed by these investigators to the 'norm' was its ability to reduce the use of clinical resources without compromising the quality of clinical care. In a subsequent publication describing the adoption of this technique in operational practice, Mintz et al. describe their analysis of data relating to pre-operative cross matching and subsequent blood use in elective surgery. Characterising local practice and generating a baseline, the authors describe the formulation and introduction of clinical practice guidelines aimed at encouraging average blood usage with reference to specific surgical procedures. Mintz et al. were able to demonstrate a substantial reduction in pre-operative cross matching and a reduction in the quantity of blood employed in some surgical operations.

Fowkes (1982) has pointed out that using a 'norm' as a clinical standard may often prove unsuccessful in precipitating a change in practice. Many clinicians, he says, will argue that divergence of their practice away from the 'norm' derives from differences in the nature and severity of illness experienced in their patients. Fernow et al. (1978) pointed out that patient variation warrants automatic consideration in clinical standard development. Again, it is interesting to note how such early thinking has led to the development of so-called 'branching' clinical guidelines which afford clinicians alternative pathways of management based on the clinical characteristics of patient presentation (see Chapter 2).

Use of clinical standards in audit: the explicit and implicit approach

Fowkes (1982) has described two methods of assessment of practice against standards; the *explicit* and *implicit* approaches. The explicit approach is characterised by direct comparison of local clinical practice with a predetermined standard of care in contrast to the implicit approach which is characterised by a comparison of local clinical practice with subjective opinion at the time of the audit. Fowkes (1982) utilises the example afforded by the work of Novick et al. (1976) in an audit of the care of paediatric iron deficiency anaemia. In this study, a panel of paediatricians formulated a set of 23 criteria which, on the basis of consensus, they considered essential elements of good clinical practice and which they agreed should be routinely recorded in the medical record. Examination of the medical records of children treated for iron deficiency anaemia was then conducted by non-medical staff to assess whether or not the agreed criteria had been satisfied in routine clinical practice. A separate panel of paediatricians employed the implicit approach in simply examining the medical records without prior knowledge of the defined criteria.

Novick *et al.* were able to report an essential similarity of the findings of the two groups, observations in agreement with the findings of independent investigators (Morehead & Donaldson 1974; Hulka *et al.* 1979).

Optimum methods in examination of clinical practice

There are, however, central considerations to be addressed in determining the optimum method for examination of clinical performance. It is noteworthy that, some 23 years ago, Brook and Appel (1973) demonstrated that audit of patient care employing the explicit method showed a less acceptable standard of patient care than when employing the implicit method in an analysis of the same patient data. The observer bias inherent in the use of the implicit method is likely to represent a prominent factor underlying this observation. Indeed, the explicit approach involves a high degree of objectivity in its analysis and by virtue of the fact that it is predetermined it cannot subsequently be modified in the judgement of the actual findings. It cannot be regarded to be completely objective, however, in that value judgements will be necessary to determine the acceptability or otherwise of identified deviations from the standard. As Fowkes (1982) points out, when clinicians are invited to make an implicit judgement of their colleagues' work, they may well be less critical than if involved in an explicit approach, with the aim, perhaps, of precluding conflict with their colleagues.

It is in this context that the value of greater objectivity is incontrovertibly clear, manifest in the ability of repeated observations of the same practice to determine definitive differences in clinical practice. This contrasts with the inherent deficiencies of the implicit approach where documented variations in clinical practice are likely to derive from variations in observer assessment. This is not to say that the explicit approach is characterised by total objectivity and a value judgement remains necessary in the examination of the acceptability of deviations from agreed clinical standards.

The explicit approach has additional benefits in that examination of practice, in terms of comparison of *actual* practice with *practice according to a given clinical standard(s)*, can be performed by non-clinical staff, given that the requirements of the standard are frequently sufficiently explicit to enable this. This therefore contrasts with the implicit approach which depends substantively on clinical interpretation and judgement and is therefore time consuming and may be considered undesirable if large numbers of patients are to be examined, that is, when patients are examined as epidemiological populations rather than as individuals. The explicit approach may sometimes require an input based on the implicit approach. In this scenario, the elements of clinical practice which may be examined appropriately by the explicit approach are examined by non-clinical staff and in those areas of practice where there are doubts about the adequacy of the explicit approach, data are examined implicitly by clinicians.

Guideline 16: Changes in clinical practice are agreed, aimed at reducing the discrepancy identified between local clinical practice and evidence-based clinical standards/guidelines/consensus statements

Changes in practice/innovations in practice agreed by the peer-review process

It is fashionable within NHS management to require evidence of change in clinical practice. Frequently, this is required as something provider units can give to purchasers as 'evidence' of clinical evaluation. There may therefore be a tendency to encourage change, simply for the sake of change. Before any practice is considered for change, it is important to invite discussions of the philosophy for change. Indeed, as Loughlin (1994) pointed out in a related context:

> 'If we hear that an ogre has given up clubbing people to death in order to write poetry, we should perhaps wait until we have actually heard the poetry before welcoming this as an unequivocal improvement.'

Changes proposed for introduction into routine clinical practice employing the mechanism of audit should therefore be highly reasoned (Guideline 11) and should derive, where possible, from a solid evidence base. Stocking (1992) is clear that proposed practice changes

> 'should be based on sound evidence, whether in terms of patients' health status or satisfaction or in terms of organisational or economic benefits to the NHS'.

Cost of changes in clinical practice

A factor of central relevance in discussions of change will be the consideration of cost. Are the practice changes proposed within the peer-review forum affordable? What is the average cost per patient of the revised treatment relative to the existing practice? While the development of clinical guidelines that form the basis of considerations of change is now proceeding with due reference to cost effectiveness as well as clinical effectiveness (Drummond 1995), it has not always done so. Guidelines being considered locally may therefore have the potential to elevate the treatment cost per patient with little corresponding increase in health gain. Where guidelines do not yet exist and local consultant consensus is employed in generating local guidelines, the same dangers can exist. The importance of strict health economic analysis in considerations of local practice change is thus clear.

Resource positive changes will need to be discussed by the medical director in his dual capacity as chairman of audit and Trust board member (Guideline 1). Such discussions will also need to take place with purchasers through the director of public health medicine in the forum of the audit steering committee (Guideline 5). A formal, standardised record of proceedings is completed at this stage and is termed the Stage 1 audit minimum data set (see p. 66). The peers agree the date for the Stage 2 outcome-evaluating audit following this Stage 1 practice-evaluating audit.

Guideline 17: Agreed changes in clinical practice are implemented with generation of process outcomes and publication of interim results

Mechanism for change implementation

Some 14 years ago, Fowkes (1982) pointed out that an audit which simply identifies deficient clinical practice may not lead to improvement in medical care. Improvement is likely only if the observation of inadequate care is followed by changes in clinical practice aimed at correcting the identified deficiency. Consensus agreement for a given change in clinical practice is one thing, implementation of that agreed change is quite another and so it is necessary to re-observe practice in order to assess whether or not any change has taken place. Implementation of change frequently fails to be achieved and in such circumstances the audit process can be seen to have generated only what Nelson (1976) has described as 'orphan data'.

In talking of the implementation of change into routine clinical practice, Fowkes considered education as a *primary* mechanism, concurrent review of practice as a *secondary* mechanism and the use of protocols as a *tertiary* mechanism. It is advanced here that a combination of these three mechanisms is vital to change implementation, rather than the use of any one such mechanism in isolation. Fowkes also employed the term *voluntary* when talking of implementing change in practice, acknowledging that 'voluntary change without any form of external sanction of incentive is difficult'. While it is clearly desirable that the changes in operational practice which are shown to be necessary by audit should be implemented through consensus and with enthusiasm this should not rule out the use of executive mandate in circumstances where change management is critical.

Take, for example, the identification by audit of inappropriate, high-risk clinical practice in a given specialty area within the organisation. Should such practices be allowed to continue, simply to avoid confrontation with the practitioner, however senior he may be, and however much held in esteem by colleagues within the organisation? Clinical risk management answers in the negative (Knowles 1995) because the circumstance discussed is not too theoretical, as any doctor or medical director will know. Obstetricians, for example, have an unfortunate association with 'unscientific practices' (see House of Commons Health Committee (1992) for examples). The exercise of such practices is medico-legally compromising and the failure to change practice based on evidence, increasingly so (Chalmers 1993; Hurwitz 1995a, b). It has also to be recognised that proposed changes in clinical practice can have benefits or disadvantages that are unrelated to patients, having greater relevance to the clinician's own security. Indeed, Lilleyman (1994) has said: 'Hell hath no fury like a vested interest paraded as a moral principle.'

In Chapter 2, Miles *et al.* describe the observation of a ten-fold increase in clinical articles employing the term 'guideline' or 'protocol' in the last decade and that in the United States, some 20 000 healthcare standards and clinical practice guidelines have been advanced by some 500 organisations. There remains, however, considerable disparity between the availability and the implementation of clinical practice guidelines. The absence of definitive methodology is central to this problem. Indeed, Treasure (1994) has said that

> 'a randomised controlled trial, however beautifully conducted, may have very little to say about how (or whether) the findings should be implemented in clinical practice – a topic of concern in the cost and audit conscious healthcare systems that most countries have these days'.

Substantial research attention has therefore focused on the methods through which agreed change can be implemented into routine clinical practice. The frequently quoted study by Georgiades and Phillimore (1975) has been followed by a multiplicity of approaches to the study and testing of single and combined methods (Stolz 1981; Rogers 1983; Fowkes *et al.* 1986a, b; Tierney *et al.* 1986; Domenighetti *et al.* 1988; Pettigrew 1988; Lomas *et al.* 1989; Lomas 1990; Lomas *et al.* 1991; Stocking 1992; Anderson *et al.* 1994; Grimshaw *et al.* 1995; Lee *et al.* 1995).

'Personal educational objectives' and change implementation

Brown and Uhl (1970) described an interesting approach to educational intervention in audit and change implementation, by encouraging doctors to formulate their own personal educational objectives based on the scale of discrepancy between their personal clinical practice and a given standard. Seminars were then forward planned as direct educational interventions aimed at improving the quality of practice. One example advanced by Brown and Uhl centred on the appropriateness of antibiotic prescribing. Clinicians were invited to complete a questionnaire on simulated case histories derived from their own personal clinical practice, with each case being subsequently considered in the forum of the organised seminar.

This approach was augmented by supporting clinical literature and by contributions from specialists in the field. Brown and Uhl were able to demonstrate a degree of modification in subsequent clinical practice, but the results of the study were disappointing and failed to demonstrate the utility of their technique in precipitating a sustained change in routine clinical practice. Several studies have generated similar results. Take, for example, the work of Achong *et al.* (1977), Jones *et al.* (1977) and Reilly and Patten (1978), who demonstrated that the simple provision of information alone is ineffective in precipitating practice changes. Newsletters and participation in workshops are similarly considered to be ineffective (Williamson *et al.* 1967), and in studies where feedback has shown a degree of effectiveness early cessation of feedback resulted in reversal of behaviour to former practices (Dombal *et al.* 1974; Rhyne & Gehlbach 1979; Verbey *et al.* 1979).

Importance of teaching method in educational intervention and change management

Robinson (1994) believes that many of the educational interventions that have been tested have not necessarily utilised the most effective teaching methods and has observed that four basic approaches to precipitating change in clinical practice have been taken:

- sending material by post
- traditional didactic lectures and presentations
- individually tailored instructions using small groups
- one-to-one contacts

Robinson is clear that of these interventions, the first is largely ineffective, the second is useful only in increasing awareness of issues (Haynes *et al.* 1984; Kosecoff *et al.* 1987; Lomas *et al.* 1989), the third appears marginally effective, but the fourth appears to be significantly effective. Robinson draws attention to the rather empirical evidence in this context that pharmaceutical marketing divisions direct funds to this approach (Soumerai *et al.* 1989). Further evidence of the importance of the one-to-one contact may be derived from the work of Coleman *et al.* (1966), Geertsma *et al.* (1982) and Greer (1988) with the work of Shaffner *et al.* (1983) and Friis *et al.* (1991) emphasising the importance of the status of the educator, and the environment in which the one-to-one educational intervention takes place.

Haines & Jones (1994) make the point that communication of ideas occurs most effectively between people who share important attributes such as educational level, belief, social status and networks. This is described as *homophily*, these authors say, with those who are advocates of clinical practice change being, or being perceived to be, *heterophilous* with the practising clinicians who mediate the adoption or rejection of recommended change (Rogers 1983). Changes in clinical practice are most likely when the educator is a doctor than if he is not (Shaffner *et al.* 1983) and when he is respected by peers (Lomas *et al.*

1991). One study of the learning environment demonstrated that recommendations for changes in antibiotic prescribing practices were more likely to be adopted when delivered by a credible source, for example a senior physician in a microbiology department, than in the fora organised by local medical societies (Friis *et al.* 1991). Some evidence exists for the utility of educational interventions by external experts to practitioners within their practice settings (Avorn *et al.* 1988; 1992; Soumerai *et al.* 1993).

The combination of direct education of clinicians with feedback (Everett *et al.* 1983; Whiteside *et al.* 1987; Mozes *et al.* 1989) may only prove effective when this approach is adopted over a protracted period of time (Harris *et al.* 1984; 1985) and with multidisciplinary involvement (Eckerlund & Jonsson 1985; Kokkola & Sintonen 1985). Analysis of the results of these studies, controlling for methodological deficiencies (Williams 1988), shows that no single strategy is likely to be successful (Stocking 1992). On the contrary, the research shows the effectiveness of an approach which combines several methodologies. This is like to be: *Direct education of clinicians by an educator whom they perceive as authoritative, in a clinical setting related to the area of practice being audited, followed by continuous feedback over an augmented period of time, with multidisciplinary involvement.*

In the method advanced in this paper, recognition of the likely effectiveness of this approach has led to the recommendation that direct education of clinicians occurs prior to the Stage 1 practice evaluating audit (Guideline 11), is provided by educators that they perceive as authoritative (Guideline 11) in an area related to the clinical practice (Guideline 11), with the results of post-audit change monitoring (Guideline 17) fed back to clinicians in continuous fashion over a protracted period of time (Guideline 17) and in a clinical setting related to the audit (Guideline 17).

When agreement for changes in clinical practice has been secured within the peer-review forum, it is necessary, as part of the implementation strategy, to consider the precise nature of the changes agreed so that it is possible to assess the nature and extent of change that is required for implementation into routine practice.

Simple, intermediate and complex categories of change in clinical practice

The peer-review forum may agree changes in practices which fall into a *simple* category, an *intermediate* category and a *complex* category. Components of change that might fall into the simple category might be the agreement to implement, for example, the standard that 90% of eligible patients admitted with a diagnosis of acute myocardial infarction should receive thrombolysis within 25 minutes of arrival in the Accident and Emergency Department. The decision may have been reached following demonstration by an audit that local practice failed to satisfy this standard. There is *one* component which constitutes the change in practice: 'Door to needle' within < 25 minutes in 90% (eligible patients). Monitoring the implementation of this change will therefore involve identifying the total sample of eligible patients, noting the 'arrival time' for each and also the 'time of initiation of thrombolysis' in that sample. The data capture form shown in Figure 4.1 would enable this.

In an intermediate category, there will be more than one component to the agreed change. Take, for example, the guidelines for management of acute myocardial infarction adopted within the South Birmingham Health Authority for clinical practice within the Reception/A&E phase:

- ECG monitoring established within 5 minutes.
- Twelve-lead ECG taken within 15 minutes.
- IV access, if not established, secured within 15 minutes.
- Pain relief given within 15 minutes.
- Decision for thrombolytic therapy reached and recorded and, if so decided, implemented within 30 minutes.

The data capture form shown in Figure 4.2 would enable a direct comparison of performance against the standards.

In a complex category, the peer-review process may have agreed to replace audit-characterised existing practice with a completely new set of clinical standards in algorithmic form. Take for example the algorithm proposed by Nee *et al.* (1994) which prescribes a complete treatment regimen for acute myocardial infarction. The methodological principles for monitoring the extent of implementation of its clinical practice standards remain the same as in the simple and intermediate categories and are fully cross applicable.

Operational implementation of practice change monitoring mechanisms

In operational terms, a statistically valid sample of new patients, whose treatment should include the agreed practice changes, is analysed a month after the Stage 1 audit which has agreed the practice changes. The clinical audit assistants, or the project managers, or collaborating clinicians (depending on the clinical complexity of the information) then directly compare what was done to the patient (medical record) with what *should* have been done to the patient (agreed changes) in each case, within the statistically valid monthly sample of new patients.

Change implementation could be defined as *complete* if all of the principal components of the agreed practice changes have been implemented, or *variably partial* if only some elements of change of the total number agreed have been introduced, in whatever combination. These data are easily illustrated in histogrammatic fashion which allows easy presentation to busy clinicians. This whole process is repeated on a monthly basis for a period of one year.

Monthly monitoring of change implementation and simple illustration of results

The findings from the monthly sampling and analysis exercise can be illustrated on a patient-to-patient basis or in aggregated fashion. It is recommended that both approaches are taken in practice. Although the illustration of such data on a patient-to-patient basis may be considered to be laborious in theory, it need not necessarily prove so in practice. Take, for example, presentations of myocardial infarction in a typical district general hospital which might number 480 per annum. A 50% sample of the monthly presentations would be represented by 20 patients. The analysis of clinical practice change implementation, in the manner described, could then easily be achieved in continuous fashion, in parallel with identification of admission through the Accident and Emergency Department. Take, in this context, the example of the South Birmingham Health Authority guidelines for management of MI (Crump 1994) and to which Figure 4.2 refers. Five definitive elements of practice change may be delineated from this detail, in the manner illustrated. When these elements of practice change are numbered formally, and when the data capture pro forma is employed (Figure 4.2) it becomes possible to monitor precisely the extent to which the elements of practice change are being completely or variably partially introduced into routine clinical practice.

Consider, for example, the following results that may be generated in a sample of 100 patients admitted with MI:

Implementation of practice changes 1–5	$(n = 60)$
Implementation of practice changes 2–5	$(n = 10)$
Implementation of practice changes 1–4	$(n = 20)$
Implementation of practice changes 1–3 and 5	$(n = 8)$
Implementation of other practice changes	$(n = 2)$

The generation of these data is essentially simple using the methodology described and can be followed by data aggregation in the manner illustrated in Figure 4.3. If this exercise is repeated on a monthly basis, the extent of change implementation can be monitored precisely and may be visualised in the manner illustrated in Figure. 4.4.

Strict deadlines need to be observed to ensure the success of the process, so the system requires that the clerical staff make raw data available four days prior to the last working day of each month. Clinical audit project managers aggregate the raw data into the categories of complete or variably partial guidelines implementation, illustrating the assimilated data in histogrammatic form, as outlined above, with a brief textual description of the findings. This information is made available to the head of department of clinical audit on the penultimate working day of each month in the forum of a personal meeting with the project managers. On the following day, the last working day of the month, the head of department of clinical audit provides these results to the relevant clinicians (within their clinics/

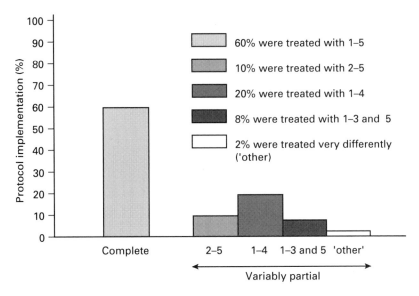

Fig. 4.3   Conceptual diagram illustrating a method for monitoring the extent of implementation into routine practice of delineated components of 'best care'.

theatres, if possible). He then meets with the chair of audit (Guideline 1) in the forum of an hour briefing meeting, during which strategic direction is given on how any identified difficulties may be quickly and effectively resolved. A principal difficulty, which may occur especially at the beginning of the prospective data collection, will be that of non-compliance with the changes agreed at the Stage 1 audit peer review session. In such cases, the chairman of audit may invite the head of department of clinical audit to hold immediate discussions with the consultant firm(s) responsible, or may elect to do so personally, depending on local circumstances and the particular characteristics of the identified deficiency.

Consideration of definitions from agreed practice changes during the implementation phase

The particular benefit of individual patient data is that identified digressions from the agreed change can be easily considered by the next peer-review forum or a working group constituted with the authority of the peers. Such an exercise is important because a particularly unusual patient may require a different method of intervention and as such would be identified by the monthly sampling described. That individual patient could then be examined by the peer review using the well-established method of case review. If the 'digression' is justified, the peers will support it. If it is not justified, then further, direct education of the treating clinician is indicated.

Deviations from the pre-existing algorithmic mode of practice that are deemed 'justified' by the peer-review group are of particular

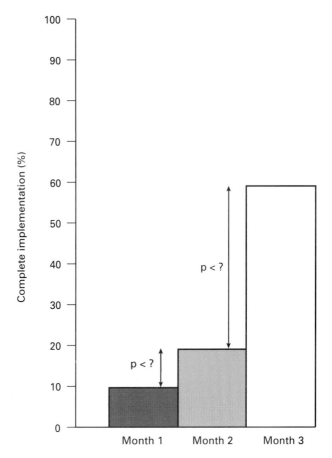

Fig. 4.4 Conceptual diagram illustrating a method for monitoring the incremental introduction of clinical guidelines into routine clinical practice.

importance in that they may demonstrate the inadequacy or limitation of existing guidelines and can be directly taken into account as part of the regular review and updating of those clinical guidelines by the Royal Colleges and other authoritative bodies.

Fundamental utility of the implementation monitoring mechanism

Through the use of this mechanism, agreed changes in practice can be introduced in incrementally increasing fashion, into routine clinical practice. This is of clear advantage to provider clinicians in shifting local practice into alignment with recommended best practice. It is of particular use to purchasers of provider services in that it represents an ideal tool through which detailed monitoring can take place. The examples of purchaser concerns described in Guideline 5 can be translated into specific standards, the introduction of which can then be monitored using the mechanism described. Provider organisations are thus empowered to provide 'hard data' on the extent of change implementation.

As purchasers move away from the purchasing of activity alone to purchase of protocols of care (Miles *et al.* 1995; Chapter 8), the availability of such data will prove of no small significance in contract negotiations with purchasers by competing provider organisations. Such data, along with associated publications, can be paired with contract prices and included in key contract negotiation documents. Here we see a further interface between clinicians and managers in the clinical audit process, and one which reinforces the interests of the other, as Bowden, writing in Chapter 10, shows.

Publication of interim results

It is particularly important to publish data deriving from audit so that a growing body of experience can be contributed to the literature for the purposes of learned review and dissemination. Publication of data deriving from implementation of evidence-based guidelines and the resulting quantified benefit provides an additional link between audit and education and has several benefits to Trust boards and purchasers. These have been outlined immediately above in terms of contract negotiation. As Margison (1994) has pointed out:

> 'the audit process often challenges received wisdom in Medicine, which itself may never have been subject to randomised controlled trials. In this situation, it is helpful to publish provisional findings, which can then be scrutinised more exactly.'

A further benefit of the publishing process is that it increases significantly the interest of junior (and consultant) medical staff in the audit process. This is particularly valuable, notably in terms of securing a high level of clinical assistance but also in directly facilitating the understanding of audit by juniors and their training in basic audit and research skills. Where the publications being written involve nurses and allied professionals, the same benefits are present and these professionals gain valuable (often initial) education in research methodology and the application of critical thought.

Potential conflicts may arise at this point with senior colleagues sitting on the Trust board. So-called 'negative' or 'bad' audit results are immediately commercially sensitive to the business planning mechanism of the Trust, and where a given Trust is in frank competition with a given provider for the maintenance of existing health contracts or the winning of new ones, it is possible that the Trust board might ask for the publication of such results to be delayed or suppressed. This is a situation which could easily compromise the medical director in his role as chairman of the clinical audit steering committee. It is highly recommended, therefore, that the process of publication is directed and managed by individual consultant firms taking part in the audit, with the support of the chairman of the appropriate audit implementation subcommittee. If difficulties emerge, the director of public health medicine and the consumer representative of the clinical audit steering committee must be approached. This course of action, if necessary, is suggested to represent an ethical and professional responsibility of the head of department of clinical audit and of his relevant clinical colleagues.

Guideline 18: Clinical audit data are presented to clinicians in Stage 2 clinical audit peer-review forum

The data accumulated during the one-year period of practice change implementation will have been analysed and process outcomes will have been generated in the manner described (Guideline 17). The methods through which definitive improvements in the outcomes of care will be demonstrated using the final pool of data at month 12 should similarly have been considered in parallel with the monthly data collection.

The process outcomes generated by the data should be illustrated in simple histogrammatic form in the Stage 2 audit peer-review forum, enabling full communication of the accumulated data. The educational benefits to junior staff that have been gained and the papers that have been written or submitted to learned clinical journals, may also be described at this time. Preliminary outcome measures may be advanced for consideration of the peers at this stage and agreement should be reached as to the direction of the final analysis and writing-up of results for publication. When such agreement has been achieved, it is likely that detailed statistical treatment of the data will be necessary and this must take place outside of the peer-review forum. Health economic analysis must also take place so that the positive, negative or neutral resource implications of the actual practice changes can be compared with those estimated and anticipated during the earlier discussion of change implementation (Guideline 16). Resource savings, when quantified, can begin forming a case for investing those monies elsewhere in the same specialty areas, for service development.

Guideline 19: Clinical benefit deriving from implementation of practice change is quantitatively measured and qualitatively described

The Royal College of Physicians (1989) has described *outcome* as follows:

> 'Outcome is the result of clinical intervention. It is considered by the College as the most relevant indicator of the quality of patient care and an essential balance to performance indicators that relate entirely to process and cost.'

The measurement of outcome following audit is the ultimate phase of the audit process and is represented by the so-called 'closing of the loop'.

Shaw (1989) makes the point that

'in some cases it is easier, and scientifically legitimate, to measure process (what is done) as a proxy for outcome (what results are achieved)'.

This approach is of greatest utility when clinical guidelines, derived from a randomised controlled trial evidence base, are available. Outcome from community immunisation programmes is similarly 'measurable' in terms of uptake and on the basis that immunisation may be presumed to precipitate immunological protection from a given disease. In absolute terms it is dangerous and scientifically untenable to believe that a given outcome will automatically result from a given process and, as Naish *et al.* (1995) point out: 'methods that link process to patient outcomes are needed before we can really talk about effectiveness'. Indeed, the relationship between process and outcome is probabilistic and not deterministic (Miles *et al.* 1995). That current methodological difficulties should not preclude even rudimentary attempts to measure outcome is supported by Evans (quote in Chalmers 1995) who has said 'it is better to measure imprecisely that which is relevant, than to measure precisely that which is irrelevant'. The attendant limitations of this approach must nevertheless be appreciated.

Long (1994) describes outcomes as the results (effects) of processes and therefore attributable to processes, though this simple definition is made subject to the emphasis that in the assessment of outcomes inputs must necessarily be measured, and among these will be patient characteristics and accurate descriptions and assessments of process elements. Also important is the need to identify any other factors separate to a given clinical indication that may be capable of precipitating observed changes, or lack of observed change. It is therefore of fundamental importance to achieve confidence that the process itself is leading *per se* to the outcome.

Measures of healthcare outcome: initial thinking

Some form of measure of outcome has always been important in healthcare. The writings of Florence Nightingale in relation to nursing triage document early thinking in this regard and focus on gross measures of patient outcome following a given medical intervention. Did the patient recover? Did the patient stay the same? Did the patient get worse? McKee (1993) has provided a conceptual model which is helpful during the initial consideration of outcome measurement (Figure 4.5) and of immediate use in this context. Holland (1983) describes negative outcome measures as death, disease, disability, discomfort and dissatisfaction. These measures are of significant utility in gross measurements of patient outcome but, as Orchard (1994; 1995) points out, none represents a satisfactory measure on its own given the multidimensional nature of clinical outcome. Indeed, Orchard (1994) emphasises that

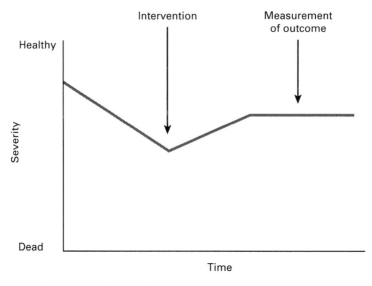

Fig. 4.5   Conceptual diagram illustrating the fundamental principle associated with measurement of outcome from clinical intervention (McKee 1993). Reproduced with permission from BMJ Publishing Group.

'the complexity of what hospitals do makes (outcome) measurement difficult, even in the narrow speciality of acute care, not least because the resources used, the choice of treatments, and the observed results are so dependent on the sorts and conditions of patients admitted – the hospital casemix'.

Long *et al.* (1993) have made the point that health service outcomes will have effects on health but will also include patient satisfaction and the attitude of patients to the services they have received within the NHS. These authors believe that what gets measured within the NHS will depend on who wants the data and for what purpose and it is likely, therefore, that the direction of outcome measurement within the NHS will be set by purchasers and clinical researchers. Long *et al.* recognised that the outcome from some services will prove considerably more difficult to measure than others and, for example, cite consultations without interventions (where the service offered has low level effects), long courses of rehabilitation or continued amelioration of symptoms in chronic illness (where the start and end of treatment are unclear) or where there is comorbidity or where several treatments are being conducted simultaneously. On the basis of this recognition, Long *et al.* advanced three prerequisites for success and meaning in the measurement of outcome:

(1)   Treatment episodes require careful definition.
(2)   Methods must exist to control for variations in patient characteristics (severity, age, comorbidity) and for service factors such as casemix, and there must be ways of isolating the effect due to the

service and those due to other factors from within and outside the health service.

(3) The period of data collection must be long enough to ensure that all relevant effects will appear or that a sufficiently large sample can be studied.

Basic methodological criteria for outcome measurement and the need for reproducibility and sensitivity

The guidelines advanced by Long *et al.* (1993) represent the basic methodological criteria for ensuring that the method used produces the same result when re-applied to the same situation. This is an absolute prerequisite of reproducibility and reliability. Such methods must measure what in fact they were designed to measure and this prerequisite ensures methodological rigour and validity. The method must also demonstrate its ability to detect change, subtle and otherwise, in the clinical parameter under investigation in order that the tool may be responsive, that is, *sensitive.*

Clinical outcome measurement

Calman (1992) is equally concerned with the principle of measuring the outcome of clinical care and sees this process as integrally linked to professional development and education, clinical audit accreditation, standards, guidelines and protocols. He understands outcome in terms of the effect of clinical intervention on the patient, family and the community as the end result of one or more episodes of care provided over a period of time for an individual. An outcome is therefore open to subjective and objective assessment by the individual, family and community and by the associated healthcare professionals. In terms of the determinants for validity of measurement of clinical outcome, Calman is in broad agreement with Long *et al.* (1993) in recognising the existence of several principal factors. Thus, Calman emphasises the need to assess:

- the health of the individual at the start of the process of care, a complex issue involving broader social dimensions such as support at home
- the illness and to be aware of the characteristics of its natural history, a need often left unrecognised, yet one which will be an important determinant of outcome
- the treatments available and to ensure the availability of details relating to their effectiveness
- the facilities and resources available.

The word 'outcome' is employed in a multiplicity of ways and in varying health service circumstances. It is widely assumed that all 'outcomes' are essentially similar, both conceptually and in terms of the manner in which they may be measured. Such a position is inherently fallacious since it is well recognised by specialists in this field that there are highly substantial differences between clinical interventions within the NHS. One may think of the differences within and between: surgical interventions, drug interventions, nursing interventions and interventions by the range of professions allied to medicine. As Hunt (1994) has pointed out,

> 'the measurement of outcome ... is profoundly problematic ... and at what point can an outcome be considered to be an outcome rather than part of a continuing process'.

This is an important point because differences in the timing of measurements can result in very different judgements about the same intervention (Hunt 1994). The author concludes that 'outcome measurement in the health services field is characterised by unsympathetic, ill-defined and unco-ordinated studies'.

Central necessity for casemix correction in outcome measurement

Rowan *et al.* (1993) have considered variation in casemix of adult admissions to general intensive care units and the impact that this factor will have on clinical outcome and its interpretation. With direct reference to such factors it is necessary to consider whether NHS Trusts with high mortality rates provide ineffective surgery or whether they admit sicker patients. Casemix, in combination with ineffective surgery, may also generate high mortality rates (Dubois *et al.* 1987) and so further controlling calculations are warranted. Indeed, adjustments for casemix frequently reduce (Green *et al.* 1991; Rowan *et al.* 1993) and can sometimes reverse (Tarnow-Mordi *et al.* 1990) *prima facie* judgements about relative performance.

Several investigators have engaged in the development of methodologies aimed at casemix correction for outcome measurement. The existing casemix systems are primarily concerned with treatments and it is clear that outcome measurement needs to be focused firmly on patients. Such a focus, as Orchard (1994) has said, requires the formulation of casemix groups that addresses both conceptual and practical difficulties in relation to:

- the nature of prognosis
- the source of patient data
- the statistical analysis of data
- the identification and weighting of patient risk factors
- the definition and measurement of severity.

For elegant discussion under each of these factors the reader is referred to Orchard (1994).

Routine data in clinical outcome measurement

Much has been written about the use of routine data for clinical audit (e.g. McKee *et al.* 1994; Williams 1995) and it is certainly true that, with given refinements and integrity checks, such routine data can prove useful in the audit process (Wyatt 1995), but the coding and recording of routine patient data within most NHS Trusts is likely to prove inadequate for use in outcome measurement (Gulliford 1992; Orchard 1994). Concerted efforts are being made to improve data integrity within the NHS (Buckland 1993; Leaning 1993) and to reduce the often alarming discrepancy between *what was done* and *what was recorded as having been done* (Wyatt 1994a–c; 1995). Until further progress has been made it is recommended that data capture, collection and integrity assurance systems are set up as part of each audit so that all interested parties can have confidence in the results.

Routine observational data which are derivable, for example, from hospital discharge summaries, are often recommended for use in measuring clinical outcome, though in many cases these data will be biased as a consequence of non-random selection of patients or treatment. Indeed, Orchard (1994) is clear that clinical decision making in relation to referrals and treatment is exercised with reference to individual prognostic assessments. Such assessments are likely to be influenced by non-medical factors in addition to considerations of disease severity, comorbidity and the anticipated effectiveness and acceptability of the intervention.

Failure to exercise control for so-called confounding factors such as age, frailty and severity can lead to spurious conclusions. Take, for example, the controversy in relation to the clinical outcomes reported for transurethral resection of prostate versus open prostatectomy for prostatic adenocarcinoma (Fisher & Wennberg 1990; Concato *et al.* 1992) and angioplasty versus coronary artery bypass grafting in severe angina (Hartz *et al.* 1992; RITA Trial Participants 1993). In both of the examples quoted, the difficulties in achieving consensus agreement in interpretation of clinical outcome data derived from the contention that age and severity had remained uncontrolled. In this context, Orchard (1994) reminds us of the dangers of one confounding variable by over-adjusting for another, giving the example of data on respiratory illness, where adjustment for cigarette smoking might mask the effects of socio-economic status.

Use of risk-adjusted observational data

The use of risk-adjusted observational data will continue to contribute to the clinical literature and to play a significant part in the debates which focus on the methodological limitations of outcome measurement techniques. Adjustment for severity is a particularly problematic exercise and involves the subjective opinion of severity made by the clinician. This in itself will influence outcome because it will form the basis of the choice and regimen of treatment. The USA has led the development of severity scoring systems although the working definition has varied and some scoring systems have been based on correlations of increasing case complexity with costs or have based severity scores on ratings for the extent of disease progression such as in cancer staging (Orchard 1994). The final stage in the audit cycle could therefore take two forms:

(1) Generation of a grand percentage describing the extent to which evidence-based practice has been introduced into routine clinical practice, with a description of what this can be expected to mean for patients treated locally. This approach would generate both a quantitative outcome measure (the percentage) and a qualitative description based on the benefits of the treatment that have been established by mega-trials and meta-analyses. Such an approach is likely to prove satisfactory to purchasers of healthcare services and is held by many to be meaningful in large measure.

(2) A quantitative and qualitative description of the actual clinical benefits that have manifested in patients locally as a result of the changes in practice that audit has driven and demonstrated to have taken place. This is methodologically problematic at the present time and the subject of ongoing research. Geographical differences in actual patient outcomes from, say, the same treatment regimen are highly likely to occur as a product of local factors, for example the extent and subdivision of ethnicity within the local population and definitive socio-economic differences within the local population, to say nothing of age, sex, morbidity and compliance. Such epidemiological concerns may be addressed through application of the best methods currently available, including an exquisitely sensitive statistical controlling of multiple variables and the possible use of census data (Botting *et al.* 1995). A formal, standardised record of the conclusion of the audit is made at this stage and is termed the Stage 2 audit minimum data set (see p. 67).

Conclusion

Both approaches to outcome measurement, whether singly or in combination, will be productive only if a sound methodological approach to audit management is taken within NHS provider units. The current system is advanced as suitable for immediate introduction into operational practice. It was judged necessary to contribute the method to the literature in full detail, though it is acknowledged that the system is complex and requires careful study prior to operational implementation with NHS provider organisations. The authors are currently preparing a simplified version, but in the interim make the point that the system is amenable to modification if necessitated by local factors such as resource limitation. For example, patient sample sizes for audit may be calculated at the threshold of statistical validity, one key element only of change in a given practice area may be examined and implementation monitoring could be performed on a quarterly, rather than monthly, basis. Functions may be shared and overall staffing levels thus reduced. Local priorities and needs will dictate the extent of modification of this methodology but they will need to preserve the fundamental prerequisites for validity that have been discussed.

Note

An abridged version of this system, as it is described in Chapters 3 and 4, was published in 1996 in the *Journal of Evaluation in Clinical Practice* (Miles *et al.* 1996b).

References

Achong, M.R., Wood, J., Theal, H.K., Goldberg, R. & Thompson, D.A. (1977) Changes in hospital antibiotic therapy after a quality-of-use study. *Lancet* **ii**: 1118–22.

Anderson, F.A., Wheeler, H.B. & Goldberg, R.J. (1994) Changing clinical practice: prospective study of the impact of continuing medical education and quality assurance programmes on the use of thromboprophylaxis in venous thromboembolism. *Annals of Internal Medicine* **154**: 669–77.

Avorn, J., Soumerai, S.B. & Taylor, W. (1988) Reduction of incorrect antibiotic dosing through a structured educational order form. *Archives of Internal Medicine* **148**: 1720–24.

Avorn, J., Soumerai, S.B. & Everitt, D.E. (1992) A randomised trial of a program to reduce the use of psychoactive drugs in nursing homes. *New England Journal of Medicine* **327**: 168–73.

Berwick, D.M. (1989) Continuous improvement as an ideal in health care. *New England Journal of Medicine* **320**: 53–6.

Black, N. & Thompson, E. (1993) Obstacles to medical audit: British doctors speak. *Social Science and Medicine* **36**: 849–56.

Botting, B., Reilly, H. & Harris, D. (1995) Use of Office of Population Censuses and Surveys records in medical research and clinical audit. *Health Trends* **27**: 4–7.

Brook, R.H. & Appel, F.A. (1973) Quality of care assessment: choosing a method of peer review. *New England Journal of Medicine* **288**: 1323–7.

Brown, C.R. & Uhl, F.A. (1970) Mandatory continuing education: sense or nonsense? *Journal of the American Medical Association* **213**: 1660–65.

Buckland, R. (1993) The language of health: a clinical language underlies the NHS information strategy. *British Medical Journal* **306**: 287–8.

Burke, C.W. (1994) Where are we? Are we going forwards or sideways? *Auditorium* **1**: 11–13.

Buttery, Y., Walshe, K., Coles, J. & Bennett, J. (1994) *Evaluating Medical Audit: The Development of Audit-Findings of a National Survey of Healthcare Provider Units in England*, CASPE Research Reports, London.

Buxton, M.J. (1994) Achievements of audit in the NHS. *Quality in Health Care* **3** (Suppl.): 531–4.

Calman, K. (1992) Quality: a view from the centre. *Quality in Health Care* **1** (Suppl.): S28–S33.

Chalmers, I. (1993) Underuse of antenatal corticosteroids and future litigation. *Lancet* **341**: 699.

Chalmers, I. (1995) What do I want from health research and researchers when I am a patient? *British Medical Journal* **310**: 1315–18.

Charlton, B.G. (1993) Management of science. *Lancet* **342**: 99–100.

Coleman, J.S., Katz, E. & Menze, L.H. (1966) *Medical Innovation: A Diffusion Study*, Bobbs-Merrill, Indianapolis, IN.

Concato, J., Horowitz, R.I., Feinstein, A.R., Elmore, J.G. & Schiff, S.F. (1992) Problems of comorbidity in mortality after prostatectomy. *Journal of the American Medical Association* **267**: 1077–82.

Crump, B. (1994) *Guidelines for Management of MI*. South Birmingham Health Authority.

Dombal, F.T., Leaper, D.J., Horrocks, J.C., Staniland, J.R. & McCann, A.P. (1974) Humans and computer-aided diagnosis of abdominal pain: further report with emphasis on performance of clinicians. *British Medical Journal* **1**: 376–80.

Domenighetti, G., Luraschi, P., Gutzwiller, F., Pedrinis, E., Casabianca, A., Spinelli, E. & Repetto, F. (1988) Effect of information campaign by the mass media on hysterectomy rates. *Lancet* **ii**: 1470–73.

Drummond, M. (1995) The role of health economics in clinical evaluation. *Journal of Evaluation in Clinical Practice* **1**: 71–5.

Dubois, R.W., Rogers, W.H., Moxley, J.H., Draper, D. & Brook, R.H. (1987) Hospital inpatient mortality. *New England Journal of Medicine* **317**: 1674–80.

Dunn, G. (1989) *Design and Analysis of Reliability Studies*, Oxford University Press, New York.

Eckerlund, I. & Jonsson, E. (1985) Economic evaluation of a Swedish medical care programme for hypertension. *Health Policy* **5**: 299–306.

Edwards, M.S.D., Fergusson, C.M. & Marshall, R.W. (1992) A change in fracture management resulting from orthopaedic audit activity. *Auditorium* **1**: 33–6.

Everett, G.C., Deblois, D., Chang, P.F. & Holle, T.S.T. (1983) Effect of cost education, cost audits and faculty chart review on the use of services. *Archives of Internal Medicine* **143**: 942–4.

Fernow, L.C., Mackie, C., McColl, I. & Rendall, M. (1978) The effect of problem-orientated medical records on clinical management controlled for patient risk. *Medical Care* **16**: 476–81.

Fisher, E.S. & Wennberg, J.E. (1990) Administrative data in effectiveness studies: the prostatectomy assessment. In: *Effectiveness and Outcomes in Healthcare* (eds K.A. Heithoff & K.N. Lohr), National Academy Press, Washington, DC.

Fowkes, F.G.R. (1982) Medical audit cycle: a review of methods and research in clinical practice. *Medical Education* **16**: 228–38.

Fowkes, F.G.R., Hall, R. & Jones, J.H. (1986a) Trial of strategy for reducing the use of laboratory tests. *British Medical Journal* **292**: 883–5.

Fowkes, F.G.R., Davies, E.R. & Evans, K.T. (1986b) Multicentre trial of four strategies to reduce use of a radiological test. *Lancet* **i**: 367–70.

Friis, H., Bro, F., Mabeck, C.E. & Vejlsgaard, F. (1991) Changes in prescription of antibiotics in general practice in relation to different strategies for drug information. *Danish Medical Bulletin* **38**: 380–82.

Gabbay, J. & Laytonj, A.J. (1992) Evaluation of audit of medical in-patient records in a district general hospital. *Quality in Health Care* **1**: 43–7.

Geertsma, R.H., Whitbourne, S.K. & Parker, R.C. (1982) How physicians view the process of change in their practical behaviour. *Journal of Medical Education* **52**: 752–61.

Georgiades, N.J. & Phillimore, L. (1975) The myth of the hero-innovator and alternative strategies for organisational change. In: *Behaviour Modification with the Severely Handicapped* (eds C. Kiernan & J. Woodford). Associated Scientific Press, USA.

Godwin, J. (1995) The importance of clinical skills. *British Medical Journal* **310**: 1281–2.

Graeme-Smith, D. (1995) Evidence-based medicine: Socratic dissent. *British Medical Journal* **310**: 1126–7.

Green, J., Passman, L.J. & Wintfield, N. (1991) Analysing hospital mortality. The consequence of diversity in patient mix. *Journal of the American Medical Association* **265**: 1849–53.

Greer, A.L. (1988) The state of the art versus the state of the science: the diffusion of new medical technologies into practice. *International Journal of Technology Assessment in Health Care* **4**: 5–26.

Grimshaw, J., Eccles, M. & Russell, I. (1995) Developing clinically valid practice guidelines. *Journal of Evaluation in Clinical Practice* **1**: 37–48.

Gulliford, M.C. (1992) Evaluating prognostic factors: implications for measurement of health care outcome. *Journal of Epidemiology and Community Health* **46**: 323–6.

Haines, A. & Jones, R. (1994) Implementing findings of research. *British Medical Journal* **308**: 1488–92.

Halliday, N. (1992) The outcome of medical audit. In: *Auditing Medical Audit*, Conference proceedings from BMA Conference 'Auditing Medical Audit', pp. 48–52.

Harris, C.M., Jarman, B. & Woodman, E. (1984) *Prescribing, a suitable care for treatment*, Occasional Paper No. 24, Royal College of General Practitioners, London.

Harris, C.M., Jarman, B. & Woodman, E. (1985) Prescribing – a case for prolonged treatment. *Journal of the Royal College of General Practitioners* **35**: 284–7.

Hartz, A.J., Kuhn, E.M., Pryor, D.B., Krakauer, H., Young, M. & Heudebert, G. (1992) Mortality after coronary angioplasty and coronary bypass surgery (the national Medicare experience). *American Journal of Cardiology* **70**: 179–85.

Haynes, R.B., Davis, D.A., McKibbon, K.A. & Tugwell, P. (1984) A critical appraisal of the efficacy of continuing medical education. *Journal of the American Medical Association* **251**: 61–4.

Heath, D.A. (1990) Random review of hospital medical records. *British Medical Journal* **300**: 651–2.

Holland, W.W. (1983) *Evaluation in Health Care*, Oxford University Press, Oxford.

Hopkins, A. (1993) *Analysis of Comments Made by Chairpersons of Medical Audit Committees in Trust Hospitals, DMUs and DHAs in England, Wales and Northern Ireland in Response to a Questionnaire Sent Out in October 1992.* Royal College of Physicians, London.

House of Commons Health Committee (1992) *Maternity Services*, HMSO, London.

Hripcsak, G., Friedman, C., Alderson, O.P., DuMouchel, W., Johnson, S.B. & Clayton, P.D. (1995) Unlocking clinical data from narrative reports: a study of natural language processing. *Annals of Internal Medicine* **122**: 681–8.

Hulka, B.S., Romm, F.J., Parkerson, G.R., Russell, I.T., Clapp, N.E. & Johnson, F.S. (1979) Peer review in ambulatory care: use of explicit criteria and implicit judgements. *Medical Care* **17** (Suppl. 3): 1–5.

Hunt, S. (1994) Outcome assessment: time for reflection. *Health Care Analysis* **2**: 151–6.

Hurwitz, B. (1995a) Clinical guidelines: proliferation and medico–legal significance. *Quality in Health Care* **3**: 37–44.

Hurwitz, B. (1995b) Clinical guidelines and the law: advice, guidance or regulation? *Journal of Evaluation in Clinical Practice* **1**: 49–60.

Institute of Medicine (1992) *Guidelines for Clinical Practice: From Development to Use*, National Academic Press, Washington, DC.

Irvine, D. & Donaldson, L. (1994) Quality and standards in healthcare. In: *Quality Assurance in Medical Care* (eds J.S. Beck, I.A.D. Bouchier & I.T. Russell), Royal Society of Edinburgh, Edinburgh.

Jones, S.R., Barks, J., Bratton, T., McCree, E., Pannel, J., Yanchik, V.A., Browne, R. & Smith, J.W. (1977) The effect of an educational program upon hospital antibiotic use. *American Journal of Medical Science* **273**: 79–83.

Klein, R. (1996) The NHS and the new scientism. *QJM* **89**: 85–7.

Knowles, D. (1995) Clinical risk management. *British Journal of Hospital Management* **53**: 291–2.

Kokkola, K. & Sintonen, H. (1985) Introducing guidelines for medical care: experience in Finland. *Hospital Health Services Review* **81**: 261–5.

Kosecoff, J., Kanouse, D.E. & Rogers, W.H. (1987) Effects of the National Institutes of Health Consensus Development Program on Physician Practice. *Journal of the American Medical Association* **258**: 2708–2713.

Leaning, M.S. (1993) The new information management and technology strategy of the NHS: person centred. *British Medical Journal* **307**: 217.

Lee, T.H., Pearson, S.D., Johnson, P.A., Garcia, T.B. & Goldman, L. (1995) Failure of information as an intervention to modify clinical management. *Annals of Internal Medicine* **122**: 434–7.

Lembcke, P.A. (1967) Evolution of medical audit. *Journal of the American Medical Association* **199**: 111–18.

Lilleyman, J.S. (1994) Clinical standards in the reformed NHS. *Archives of Diseases in Childhood* **71**: 275–6.

Lomas, J. (1990) Promoting clinical policy change: using the art to promote the science in medicine. In: *Economic Issues in Healthcare: The Challenges of Medical Practice Variations* (eds T.T. Anderson & G. Mooney), Macmillan, Basingstoke.

Lomas, J., Anderson, G.M. & Domnick-Pierre, K. (1989) Do practice guidelines guide practice? The effect of a consensus statement on the practice of physicians. *New England Journal of Medicine* **321**: 1306–1311.

Lomas, J., Enkin, M. & Anderson, G.M. (1991) Opinion leaders vs audit and feedback to implement practice guidelines. Delivery after previous Caesarian section. *Journal of the American Medical Association* **265**: 2202–2207.

Long, A.F. (1994) Guidelines, protocols and outcomes. *International Journal of Healthcare Quality Assurance* **7**: 4–7.

Long, A.F., Dixon, P., Hall, R., Carr-Hill, R.A. & Sheldon, T.A. (1993) The outcome agenda: contribution of the UK clearing house on health outcomes. *Quality in Health Care* **2**: 49–52.

Loughlin, M. (1994) The poverty of management. *Health Care Analysis* **2**: 135–9.

Margison, F. (1994) Assessing change through audit. *British Medical Journal* **309**: 671.

McColl, I. (1979) Medical audit in British hospital practice. *British Journal of Hospital Medicine* **22**: 485–9.

McKee, M. (1993) Routine data – a resource for clinical audit? *Quality in Health Care* **2**: 104–11.

McKee, M., Dixon, J. & Chenet, L. (1994) Making routine data adequate to support clinical audit. *British Medical Journal* **309**: 1246–7.

Miles, A. (1995a) Critical inquiry into clinical practice. *Journal of Evaluation in Clinical Practice* **1**: 3–4.

Miles, A. (1995b) Purchasing quality in clinical practice: what on earth do we mean? *Journal of Evaluation in Clinical Practice* **1**: 81–4.

Miles, A., Bentley, D., Grey, J.E. & Polychronis, A. (1995) Purchasing quality in clinical practice: what on earth do we mean? *Journal of Evaluation in Clinical Practice* **1**: 87–95.

Miles, A., Bentley, D.P., Polychronis, A., Price, N. & Grey, J.E. (1996a) Clinical audit in the National Health Service: fact or fiction? *Journal of Evaluation in Clinical Practice* **2**: 29–35.

Miles, A., Bentley, D.P., Price, N., Polychronis, A., Grey, J.E. & Asbridge, J.E. (1996b) The Total Healthcare Audit System: a systematic methodology for auditing the totality of patient care. *Journal of Evaluation in Clinical Practice* **2**: 37–64.

Mintz, P.D., Lauenstein, K., Hume, J. & Henry, J.B. (1978) Expected haemotherapy in elective surgery. A follow-up. *Journal of the American Medical Association* **239**: 623–9.

Morehead, M.A. & Donaldson, R. (1974) Quality of clinical management of disease in comprehensive neighbourhood health centres. *Medical Care* **12**: 301–306.

Mozes, B., Lubin, D. & Modan, B. (1989) Evaluation of an intervention aimed at reducing inappropriate use of perioperative blood coagulation tests. *Archives of Internal Medicine* **149**: 1836–8.

Naish, J., Sturdy, P., Griffiths, C. & Toon, P. (1995) Appropriate prescribing in asthma. *British Medical Journal* **310**: 1472.

Nee, P.A., Gray, A.J. & Martin, A.M. (1994) Audit of thrombolysis initiated in an accident and emergency department. *Quality in Health Care* **2**: 29–33.

Nelson, A.R. (1976) Orphan data and the unclosed loop: a dilemma in PSRO and medical audit. *New England Journal of Medicine* **295**: 617–20.

Novick, L.F., Dickinson, K., Asnes, R., May-lan, S.P. & Lowenstein, R. (1976) Assessment of ambulatory care: application of the tracer methodology. *Medical Care* **14**: 1–6.

Orchard, C. (1994) Comparing health outcomes. *British Medical Journal* **308**: 1493–6.

Orchard, C. (1995) Measuring healthcare outcomes. *Focus on Outcome Analysis* **1**: 3–6.

O'Neill, D., Miles, A. & Polychronis, A. (1996) Central dimensions in clinical practice evaluation: efficiency, appropriateness and effectiveness I. *Journal of Evaluation in Clinical Practice* **2**: 13–27.

Parillo, J.E. (1995) Visions of the past and future: the Presidential address from the 24th Educational and Scientific Symposium of the Society of Critical Care Medicine. *Critical Care Medicine* **23**: 607–12.

Pettigrew, A. (1988) *The Management of Strategic Change*. Blackwell Science, Oxford.

Polychronis, A., Miles, A. & Bentley, D.P. (1996a) Evidence-based medicine: Reference? Dogma? Neologism? New orthodoxy? *Journal of Evaluation in Clinical Practice* **2**: 1–30.

Polychronis, A., Miles, A. & Bentley, D.P. (1996b) The protagonists of evidence-based medicine: arrogant, seductive and controversial. *Journal of Evaluation in Clinical Practice* **2**: 9–12.

Reilly, P.M. & Patten, M.P. (1978) An audit of prescribing by peer review. *Journal of the Royal College of General Practitioners* **28**: 525–31.

Rhyne, R.L. & Gehlbach, S.H. (1979) Effects of an educational feedback strategy on physician utilisation of thyroid function tests. *Journal of Family Practice* **8**: 1003–1008.

Rigge, M. (1995a) Users' involvement in clinical audit. *Journal of Evaluation in Clinical Practice* **1**: 67–70.

Rigge, M. (1995b) Whose outcome is it anyway? In: *Outcomes into Clinical Practice* (ed. T. Delamother), British Medical Journal Publishing Group, London, pp. 40–48.

RITA Trial Participants (1993) Coronary angioplasty versus coronary artery bypass surgery: the randomised intervention treatment of angina (RITA) trial. *Lancet* **341**: 573–80.

Robinson, M.B. (1994) Evaluation of medical audit. *Journal of Epidemiology and Community Health* **48**: 435–40.

Rogers, B. (1983) *Diffusion of Innovation*, 3rd ed. Free Press, New York.

Ross, P. (1992) Medical audit: a consultant's view. In: *Auditing Medical Audit*, BMA Conference Proceedings, 'Auditing Medical Audit', pp. 48–52.

Rowan, K.M., Kerr, J.H., Major, E., McPherson, K., Short, A. & Vessey, M.P. (1993) Intensive Care Society's APACHE II study in Britain and Ireland I: variations in casemix of adult admissions to general intensive care units and impact on outcome. *British Medical Journal* **307**: 972–7.

Royal College of Physicians (1989) *Medical audit – A First Report: What, Why and How?* Royal College of Physicians, London.

Royal College of Physicians (1993) *Medical Audit: A Second Report*, Royal College of Physicians, London.

Sanzaro, P.J. (1974) Medical audit. Experience in the USA. *British Medical Journal* **1**: 271–6.

Shaffner, W., Ray, W.A., Federspiel, C.F. & Miller, W.O. (1983) Improving antibiotic prescribing in office practice: a controlled trial of three educational methods. *Journal of the American Medical Association* **250**: 1728–32.

Shaw, C. (1989) *Medical Audit – A Hospital Handbook*, King's Fund Centre, KFC 89/11, London.

Soumerai, S.B., McLaughlin, T.J. & Avorn, J. (1989) Improving drug prescribing in primary care: a critical analysis of the experimental literature. *Milbank Quarterly* **67**: 268–317.

Soumerai, S.B., Salem-Schatz, S. & Avorn, J. (1993) A controlled trial of educational outreach to improve blood transfusion practice. *Journal of the American Medical Association* **270**: 961–6.

Sprent, P. (1993) *Applied Non-Parametric Statistical Methods*, 2nd ed. Chapman and Hall, London.

Stocking, B. (1992) Promoting change in clinical care. *Quality in Health Care* **1**: 56–60.

Stolz, S.B. (1981) Adoption of innovations from applied behavioural research: does anybody care? *Journal of Applied Behaviour Analysis* **14**: 491–505.

Tanenbaum, S. (1995) Getting there from here: evidentiary quandaries of the US outcomes movement. *Journal of Evaluation in Clinical Practice* **2**: 97–103.

Tarnow-Mordi, W., Ogston, S., Wilkinson, A.R., Reid, E., Gregory, J., Saeed, M. & Wilkie, R. (1990) Predicting death from initial disease severity in very low birthweight infants: a method for comparing the performance of neonatal units. *British Medical Journal* **300**: 1611–14.

Thomson, R.G. & Barton, A.G. (1994) Is audit running out of steam? *Quality in Health Care* **3**: 225–9.

Tierney, W.M., Hiu, S.L. & McDonald, C.J. (1986) Delayed feedback of physician performance versus immediate reminders to perform preventive care. *Medical Care* **24**: 659–66.

Treasure, T. (1994) From research to practice. *Lancet* **344**: 417–18.

Verbey, J.E., Holden, P. & Davies, R.H. (1979) Peer review of consultation in primary care: the use of audiovisual recordings. *British Medical Journal* **1**: 1686–91.

Whiteside, M.E., Lefkowitz, S., Justinani, F.R. & Ratzan, K. (1987) Changing practice patterns: a program of physician education. *Hospital Formulary* **22**: 561–8.

Williams, J.G. (1995) Making routine data adequate to support clinical audit: 'routine' is inadequately defined. *British Medical Journal* **310**: 665.

Williams, J.I. (1988) A taxonomy and critical review of tested strategies for the application of clinical practical recommendations. *American Journal of Preventative Medicine* **4** (Suppl.): 95–7.

Williamson, J.W., Alexander, M. & Miller, G.E. (1967) Continuing education and patient care research. Physician response to screening test results. *Journal of the American Medical Association* **201**: 188–221.

Wyatt, J.C. (1994a) Clinical data systems: data and medical records. *Lancet* **344**: 1543–7.

Wyatt, J.C. (1994b) Clinical data systems: components and techniques. *Lancet* **344**: 1609–14.

Wyatt, J.C. (1994c) Clinical data systems: development and evaluation. *Lancet* **344**: 1682–8.

Wyatt, J.C. (1995) The centrality of data adequacy and integrity in clinical practice evaluation. *Journal of Evaluation in Clinical Practice* **1**: 15–27.

Yerushalmy, J. (1969) The statistical assessment of the variability in observer perception and description of roentgenographic pulmonary shadows. *Radiology Clinics of North America* **7**: 381–92.

5 ◆ Increasing the Effectiveness of Clinical Intervention

Andrew Haines, Nick Freemantle, Ian Watt and Myriam Lugon

Introduction

There is increasing interest in interventions to promote clinical effectiveness and the transition of research evidence into practice. There is a number of reasons why clinical effectiveness is perceived as being of importance including: increasing pressure on health services to keep up with technological advances and demographic changes within limited resources; evidence that clinicians do not necessarily practise in accordance with evidence from well designed studies; and growing demands from an increasingly sophisticated public for more information about the outcomes of specific interventions. Many studies examine the efficacy of a specific intervention. This is the ability of an intervention to produce the desired outcome in a defined population under ideal conditions. It should be distinguished from the concept of effectiveness which is the extent to which that outcome is achieved under the usual conditions of care in which skills and resources may be different from those in the experimental situation.

Until recently it has been difficult for busy clinicians to obtain reliable information about the effectiveness of specific interventions in an easily digestible form. Significant developments are now occurring which should improve the situation by making widely available systematic reviews of the research evidence for a wider range of interventions (see Appendix).

Systematic reviews

It has been shown that traditional review articles have frequently been inadequate and misleading because they do not systematically include all evidence on a specific topic (Mulrow 1987). This, together with concerns about the inadequate statistical power of many individual trials, has given added impetus to the use of systematic reviews, meta-analyses and setting up of large, simple, randomised trials. Systematic reviews are being co-ordinated through the Cochrane Collaboration (Chalmers *et al.* 1992) on an ongoing bias and through the NHS Reviews and Dissemination Centre. Criteria for judging the quality of review articles have been developed (Oxman 1994). In particular it is necessary to ensure that sources of bias have been clearly identified and that methods for protecting against bias have been used. The sources of bias and methods of protection against bias are as follows:

(1) Problem formulation
- is the question clearly focused?
(2) Study identification
- is the search for relevant studies thorough?
(3) Study selection
- are the inclusion criteria appropriate?
(4) Appraisal of studies
- is the validity of included studies adequately assessed?
(5) Data collection
- is missing information obtained from investigators?
(6) Data synthesis
- how sensitive are the results to changes in the way the review is done?
(7) Interpretation of results
- do the conclusions flow from the evidence that is reviewed?
- are judgments about preferences (values) explicit?
- if there is 'no evidence of effect', is caution taken not to interpret this as 'evidence of no effect'?
- Are subgroup analyses interpreted cautiously?

Oxman (1994)

In cases where trials have included similar kinds of patients and where similar outcome measures have been used, a formal meta-analysis can assist in reaching conclusions. Such analyses need to take into account the methodological quality of the trials used and undertake sensitivity analyses which test the robustness of the results. For example, the sensitivity analysis can examine the impact on the conclusions of removing trials of lower methodological quality or of excluding unpublished studies. Meta-analyses, where there is significant heterogeneity between trials, should incorporate an investigation of the possible causes, which may include differences in the severity of the underlying disease, and extent, duration and type of the intervention (Thompson 1994). In the absence of a biased selection of studies, the reduction in events in the smaller trials should be scattered relatively symmetrically around the estimate(s) from large trial(s). This can be used to check for the possibility of publication bias caused by the failure of negative studies to be published (Eager & Davey-Smith 1995). Miles *et al.*, writing in Chapter 2, have examined the process of meta-analysis in some detail and the reader is referred to that text for further discussion.

Systematic reviews have also examined the broad questions of the effectiveness of methods to influence the delivery of healthcare. For example, the effectiveness of continuing medical education, broadly speaking (Davis *et al.* 1992) and computerised decision aids (Johnson *et al.* 1994) have been established at least in certain forms and contexts of care. However, more focused systematic reviews of the effectiveness of specific interventions (such as audit and feedback in different forms) or in different areas of clinical activity (e.g. attempts to modify prescribing behaviour) are currently lacking.

A further problem of traditional review articles published in clinical journals is that these may quickly go out of date, particularly in an area such as professional behaviour change where both new publications and existing but previously unlocated evaluations frequently appear. For these reasons the Cochrane Collaboration on Effective Professional Practice (CCEPP) has been formed to undertake systematic reviews in the area of professional behaviour change and delivery of health services (Freemantle *et al.*, 1995).

The focus of CCEPP is on reviews of interventions designed to improve professional practice and the delivery of effective health services. This includes various forms of continuing education, quality assurance, informatics, and financial, organisational and regulatory interventions that can affect the ability of healthcare professionals to deliver services more effectively or efficiently. Reviews in a number of areas are currently under development and will be made available on the Cochrane Database of Systematic Reviews, distributed by the BMJ group.

Cochrane review groups provide focus and support for researchers around the world who are interested in specific areas, and ensure that reviews which are published are of high quality and regularly updated. Cochrane reviews are made available on the Cochrane Database and build on the blueprint developed by reviewers in the area of pregnancy and childbirth (Chalmers *et al.* 1992), themselves influenced by an English epidemiologist, Archie Cochrane, who actively promoted the development of more systematic methods to review and synthesise research findings more than 20 years ago (Cochrane 1972).

Sources of information about effective treatment

There is a range of sources of information about effective interventions and a growing number of systematic reviews and meta-analyses are being published in medical journals. More conveniently, for the busy clinician, the systematic reviews are being widely disseminated by a number of agencies. In the UK, the NHS Reviews and Dissemination Centre publishes *Effective Health Care*, a bulletin on the effectiveness of health service interventions. This includes systematic reviews of the evidence on specific topics using three principle criteria: clinical effectiveness, cost effectiveness and acceptability. It also publishes other sources of information about effective treatment including *Effectiveness Matters*, which mainly summarises the results from rigorous primary research and systematic reviews not commissioned or undertaken by the centre. The database *Effective Care in Pregnancy and Childbirth* is now available on disc and regularly updated (Cochrane Collaboration 1993). A subscription issue of disc-based versions of the

Cochrane Database of Systematic Reviews across a range of topics is available. This includes all registered or prospective entities within the Cochrane Collaboration (collaborative review groups, methods groups and Cochrane centres) and a bibliography of existing reports of systematic reviews.

In the USA, the Agency for Health Care Policy and Research has developed and widely disseminated guidelines on a number of topics. Three forms of guidelines are available on each topic: a patient guide, a quick reference guide and a more complete guide that summarises the research rationale behind the guidelines. The latter is the product in part of a systematic review of research evidence (Van Amringe & Shannon 1992). The American College of Physicians (ACP) journal club includes structured reports of trials and systematic reviews.

Evidence for unacceptable delays in implementation of research findings

A number of studies has shown that clinically effective interventions have been inadequately used by health professionals. A well known example is that of thrombolytic therapy for myocardial infarction for which there was a 13-year delay between the demonstration of effectiveness from cumulative meta-analysis of randomised trials and recommendation of the treatment by most authors of review articles or book chapters (Antman *et al.* 1992). Other examples include inadequate use of steroids in women in premature labour, despite good evidence of their beneficial effect on fetal lung surfactant (Donaldson 1992). A survey of obstetric units, published in 1993, showed that systematic overviews of evidence-based practice were not well disseminated at that time, with nearly three-quarters of the obstetric units surveyed not having access to a copy of the database of obstetric trials (Patterson-Brown *et al.* 1993).

There is also evidence that some inappropriate procedures become widely disseminated without adequate evaluation. For example, William Osler supported the concept of blood-letting for the treatment of lobar pneumonia. J. Marion Sims, a prominent American gynaecologist developed the postcoital test which was intended to evaluate the ability of sperm to survive and penetrate cervical mucus. The test has been extensively adopted but has poor predictive power (Grimes 1993). Ineffective interventions may continue to be used long after their inappropriateness has been demonstrated, such as in the case of D&C in young women (Coulter *et al.* 1993).

Factors which may affect the promotion of clinical effectiveness

There are a number of major 'players' who need to be influenced or can act as influencers in trying to promote change. They are:

- individual health professionals and managers
- purchasing organisations
- provider organisations
- professional bodies, e.g. Royal Colleges
- education providers
- research information providers, e.g. NHS Centre for Reviews and Dissemination
- researchers
- public
- patients and users
- media
- 'alliance' partners, e.g. local authorities
- policy makers.

Clearly, individual health professionals are the key group to be influenced, but there are many ways in which such influence may be felt. Entities which may be powerful influences, such as professional bodies and purchasing authorities, are also themselves subject to influences from, for instance, the Department of Health or the mass media. Opinion leaders within organisations may play a key role in changing organisational policy. Levers for change include financial or contractual mechanisms to promote uptake of evidence-based practice, statutes or regulations to promote change and professional incentives or removal of disincentives.

Incentives might include questions on critical appraisal or evidence-based medicine in professional examinations or using the degree to which research evidence is implemented as one of the factors to be monitored in performance management systems. Chapters 3 and 4 of this volume describe a method with no small utility in this regard. There are several barriers to improving clinical effectiveness which include:

- lack of accessible information on effective interventions
- failure of clinicians to receive such information
- failure to act on information received
- existence of disincentives to change (e.g. financial disincentives)
- lack of clear management mechanisms to promote and maintain appropriate changes in practice
- public perceptions of appropriateness of interventions (which may not accord with the best available evidence).

The reasons for failure of many health professionals to respond to information about effectiveness are likely to be complex. Part of the problem may be information overload. It is clearly impossible for clinicians to keep up with information in over 20 000 medical journals which contain over 2 000 000 articles annually. If piled one on top of another, these would rise to five hundred metres in height (Mulrow 1994). There are also professional barriers to change in that evidence from trials may conflict with traditionally held beliefs. This challenge to received wisdom may be seen as a threat by professional organisations. The concept of evidence-based medicine is only just beginning to make an impact on programmes of undergraduate, postgraduate and continuing education.

There are frequently no incentives to keep up to date and to use interventions of proven clinical effectiveness. Sometimes there may be a disincentive, such as the need to learn a new procedure or where a new intervention may result in a loss of income for the individual practitioner (in fee for service medical systems), of the provider unit. Patient demand may fuel the use of inappropriate procedures and in turn may be influenced by the media and by deep-seated cultural beliefs. The National Health Service has no clear management mechanisms for promoting clinical effectiveness. Decision makers often set a bad example by implementing major changes in policy on largely ideological grounds, without considering evidence of effectiveness. Potential interventions which could be used are as follows:

- clinical guidelines
- audit and feedback
- conferences
- outreach visits ('academic detailing')
- local consensus processes
- educational approaches
- marketing
- opinion leaders/change agents
- reminders/computerised decision support
- patient-mediated interventions
- multifaceted interventions.

Thus, for instance, clinical guidelines could be used in a number of ways to influence some of the key players. In the USA, for example, the Agency for Health Care Policy in Research has disseminated its guidelines very widely and news of the pain guideline made the front page of 11 newspapers, was covered by at least 44 television stations and ten news programmes, and broadcast by more than 4400 radio stations (Van Amringe & Shannon 1992). More conventionally, guidelines can be developed and disseminated by professional bodies and organisations to individual health professionals and form the subject of educational programmes.

Opinion leaders in a social system influence the attitudes and behaviour of others. They tend to be respected for their technical competence and have greater exposure to external sources of information than other members of the social system. Change agents, however, are not usually members of the social system to be influenced, but work to promote the uptake of innovations. They try to make individuals aware of their need to change, provide appropriate support and information and promote continued adherence. They often use opinion leaders to promote the desired innovation.

Academic detailing is the transmission of information to

practitioners based on the activities undertaken by pharmaceutical companies' sales representatives. They have clear educational and behavioural objectives and use concise materials with positive feedback and reinforcement of the message. Fuller discussions of these roles are given elsewhere (Rogers 1983; Goldberg *et al.* 1994).

The characteristics of the 'message' may influence its uptake. For instance research findings can be presented in a number of ways – in the case of an intervention trial, relative risk (RR), relative risk reduction (RRR), absolute risk reduction (ARR) and number needed to treat (NNT) to prevent an event are all possibilities. There is evidence that the method and completeness of reporting trial results may affect doctors' willingness to use results of trials (Bobbio *et al.* 1994). Some journals are now requesting that both relative and absolute reduction are specified in reports and the ACP journal club attempts to include RRR, ARR and NNT in all abstracts about treatments (Guyatt *et al.* 1995). The NNT is becoming increasingly accepted as a useful way of giving clinicians and patients an indication of the likely benefit of a specific intervention.

Conceptual framework for the uptake of innovations

Studies of a range of sectors have shown an S-shaped curve of adoption of an innovation over time. The curve takes off after around 10–25% of the target population adopts that innovation. This is probably because opinion leaders within the group in question have taken up the innovation and rapidly transmit it to the majority of those remaining (Rogers 1983).

Of course, the slope of the S-shaped curve which reflects the rate of uptake of an innovation over time varies according to the innovation studied. A recent example from the health sector in which the rate of use of laparoscopic cholecystectomy was studied in the US State of Pennsylvania demonstrated that it took three years for the technique to be taken up by surgeons in the state (Fendrick *et al.* 1994). A number of characteristics of innovations as perceived by those to whom they are relevant may help to account for their different rates of adoption.

(1) Relative advantage is the degree to which an innovation is perceived as better than the approach which it supersedes. It is the perception of advantage from the perspective of the health professional which is likely to be of key importance. Increasingly, as the concepts of critical appraisal and evidence-based medicine become prevalent in medical culture, the perception of relative advantage should become governed by evidence of clinical effectiveness from well-designed trials.

(2) Compatibility is the extent to which an innovation is considered to be consistent with the existing values and previous experience of potential implementors. If an idea is not compatible with prevalent norms within a given social group, it may not be taken up.

On occasions changing norms and beliefs permit the rapid uptake of an innovation.

(3) The complexity of an innovation is the degree to which it is perceived as being difficult to understand and to implement. Those that are easier to understand are likely to be more rapidly taken up by a given social system.

(4) Trialability indicates the degree to which an innovation may be tested on a limited basis by those who might adopt it. This gives the potential adopters an opportunity to try out the innovation without making any lasting commitment which might involve considerable expenditure of time and resources.

(5) Observability describes the extent to which the results of an innovation are easily perceived by potential adopters. The easier it is for them to see the results of a particular innovation, the more likely they are to adopt it.

The process by which an innovation is communicated through certain channels over time to members of a social system has been called diffusion. The communication channels which can be used may be interpersonal or involve mass media. Communication is more likely to occur between those who share a range of attributes, such as beliefs, education and social status. Miles *et al.*, writing in Chapter 4, quote Haines and Jones (1994) in describing this phenomenon as 'homophily'. This may be a problem in the communication of medical advances as researchers and practitioners are frequently quite dissimilar in their backgrounds. Researchers rarely consider how best to implement the findings of their own work, and may not be well equipped to do so.

The process through which an individual moves from first knowledge about innovation to implementation and confirmation of change of practice has been considered to have five main steps (Rogers 1983). Knowledge about a new innovation (step 1) is the first of these and, in the case of medical education, knowledge has all too often been equated with a change in practice. The availability of knowledge is clearly determined by the communication channels to which the individual or unit has access. Information overload may be as great a problem as lack of information. In persuasion (step 2), the individual forms an attitude towards the innovation depending on the five perceived characteristics of the innovation given earlier. Decision making (step 3) may result in adoption or rejection of the innovation. This initial response may, of course, later be reversed in the light of experience or new evidence. Implementation (step 4) occurs when the innovation is put to use, but it may not be implemented in precisely the form in which it has been transmitted. For instance, clinicians may reinvent an innovation, either modifying it – such as in the case of surgical technique – or applying it to patient groups for which it was not intended. Finally, confirmation (step 5) occurs when the innovation becomes established because the individual or unit decides that the innovation is, indeed, appropriate practice. Interventions aimed at promoting implementation need to take into account the complexity of the process of change.

Clinical practice guidelines

Much of the work on methods of promoting clinical effectiveness in the health system has been undertaken using guidelines. Clinical practice guidelines are one way in which the findings of rigorous research and systematic reviews may be made available to those whose decisions impact upon the delivery of healthcare. Clinicians in different professional groups and sectors in health systems, managers and the commissioners of care (e.g. Health Maintenance Organisations, managers in the US, or health authorities in their commissioning function in the UK) may all have a role in the development and implementation of clinical practice guidelines. One of the potential advantages of guidelines is that they may specify the appropriate form of care where this involves collective action of a number of professionals, or where appropriate care may only be achieved through co-operation between primary and secondary care.

The uptake of research findings often requires more than a change in the behaviour of a single health professional. An example of this may be the changes required in the delivery of care to ensure prompt delivery of thrombolysis to patients with confirmed myocardial infarction (MI). There is considerable evidence to demonstrate the effectiveness of thrombolysis in reducing mortality due to acute myocardial infarction (Fibrinolytic Therapy Trialists Group 1994). However, the benefits of thrombolysis decline rapidly as the time between the onset of symptoms and therapy increases. The effectiveness of this intervention is therefore directly affected by the efficiency with which it is delivered to eligible patients, in terms of the interval between diagnosis of MI and initiation of thrombolysis (see Chapter 4).

Achieving prompt thrombolysis may require major changes in the way health services are delivered. When patients with acute MI present in primary care their symptoms must be recognised and steps taken to achieve rapid access to care. While this might normally mean ensuring rapid transfer to an acute facility, other solutions are available such as appropriately trained and equipped GP treatment in the community in rural areas (Anonymous 1992), or even mobile paramedic treatment in appropriately equipped ambulances. Even when patients are transferred to hospital substantial changes may be required to ensure prompt delivery of care. For example, it has been shown that giving thrombolytic drugs in coronary care units may delay access to treatment (Birkhead 1992), though developing an efficient triage system (likely to involve a range of accident and emergency staff including doctors, nurses and ambulance staff) may reduce delays.

Guidelines in an area such as thrombolysis may be used to promote evidence-based changes in the provision of health services where the impact of such therapy is not self-evident to health professionals in practice, for example small, but clinically important, benefits from therapies. Guidelines on their own are, however, unlikely to lead to significant improvements in the way health services are delivered.

In a systematic review of 91 evaluations of the implementation of guidelines those which were not accompanied by active implementation strategies were found to be unlikely to effect change (Nuffield Institute for Health 1994). This review located evaluations of guidelines implementation which involved medical staff through rigorous searches of the available literature, including Medline, Embase, SIGLE and DHSS-DATA. Published bibliographies of related topics were also consulted, along with the reference lists of articles reviewed and other more opportunistic methods. One of the difficulties in identifying literature in this area is that relevant articles are spread among many different journals, addressing a wide variety of clinical areas and questions on the delivery of services and there are no subject headings available in the main databases which allow coded searches.

The review found that the way in which guidelines are developed, implemented and monitored influences the likelihood of adherence to them in clinical practice. The review did not support the commonly held notion that the involvement of end users in the development of guidelines necessarily led to greater adherence. In fact the four studies which directly examined this question provided equivocal results, with two studies not supporting this hypothesis (Sommers *et al.* 1984; Putnam & Curry 1989). Of far greater importance was the manner in which guidelines were implemented. Very few evaluations in which dissemination of guidelines was limited to direct mailing or publication of guidelines in journals showed positive effects on professional behaviour.

Educational strategies, such as educational outreach visits and the use of local opinion leaders, were shown to be effective in some evaluations. Similarly, implementation strategies such as the restructuring of medical records, patient-specific reminders during consultations and patient-mediated interventions (in which the aim is to affect professional practice through informing patients) were all seen to be effective in certain circumstances. There was some evidence that educational interventions which involved active professional participation and implementation strategies that are closely related to clinical decision making are more likely to lead to successful guidelines implementation. In other words, implementation strategies which are nearer the end user and integrated into the process of healthcare delivery are more likely to be effective based on available evidence. However, limitations of the evidence reviewed prevented clear conclusions on the effectiveness of different implementation strategies in different contexts.

If guidelines contain the message on the delivery of healthcare, it is important that this is based upon good evidence of both clinical effectiveness and cost effectiveness. Very few of the guidelines reviewed were explicitly based on such evidence. Some guidelines are based upon the products of expert panels, or using methods such as the RAND appropriateness method to produce detailed criteria for intervention in the absence of research evidence. This approach was severely criticised in a recent US Congressional Office of Health Technology Assessment Report, which stated:

> Evidence based clinical practice guidelines have proved workable and politically acceptable. In fact, the theoretical strength of such guidelines is so compelling that it calls into question the usefulness of federally sponsored guidelines not based on an explicit review of evidence that considers, in some explicit and systematic fashion, the strength of that evidence. Guidelines with less evidence base may be justified for some purposes (e.g. guidance on the use of very new technologies) but those purposes should be carefully thought out.
>
> (OTA 1994, 169)

Put simply, systematising care through the implementation of guidelines which are not based upon good evidence of effectiveness and cost effectiveness may do more harm than good. Recommendations for the appraisal of guidelines have been made (Cluzeau *et al.* 1994). The desirable attributes of clinical practice guidelines are given in the list below.

(1) Validity: correctly interpreting available evidence so that, when followed, valid guidelines lead to improvements in health.
(2) Cost effectiveness: guidelines lead to improvements in health at acceptable cost.
(3) Reproducibility: given the same evidence, another guideline group produces similar recommendations.
(4) Reliability: given the same clinical circumstances, another health professional applies them similarly.
(5) Representative development: all key disciplines and interests (including patients) contribute to guideline development.
(6) Clinical applicability: target population is defined in accordance with scientific evidence.
(7) Clinical flexibility: guidelines identify exceptions and indicate how patient preferences are to be incorporated in decision making.
(8) Clarity: guidelines use precise definitions, unambiguous language, and user-friendly formats.
(9) Meticulous documentation: guidelines record participants, assumptions and methods, and link recommendations to available evidence.
(10) Scheduled review: guidelines state when and how they are to be reviewed.

(11) Utilisation review: guidelines indicate ways in which adherence to recommendations can be sensibly monitored.

Effective Health Care (Nuffield Institute for Health 1994).

Properly implemented clinical practice guidelines are one potential method for promoting evidence-based practice. However, they are not appropriate for every clinical circumstance. This is partly because of the paucity of good evidence on the effectiveness of many health technologies, and partly because even well-evaluated technologies are only worth developing and implementing if the resultant changes in clinical practice and patient benefits are worth the costs involved. The scientific basis of guideline derivation, their cost effectiveness and the methods for their implementation into routine clinical practice have been considered in Chapters 2–4.

The policy environment

Although there is some uncertainty about the specific methods and mechanisms by which clinical effectiveness can be improved, this need not act as a barrier to action. There is sufficient information available to provide a sound evidence base for policy formulation.

National responsibilities

A major central responsibility is to create a supportive policy environment in which clinical effectiveness is seen as an important health service priority. If effectiveness is not placed high on health professionals' agendas it is unlikely that practice will be influenced, particularly as in the NHS there are so many competing managerial demands. Until recently, the political and economic realities of UK healthcare and the strong financial agendas of managers (Pollitt *et al.*, 1992) have served to make efficiency the dominant indicator of quality in the NHS. However, recent directives from the NHS Management Executive (NHSME 1993; 1994) have stressed the importance of clinical effectiveness and identified its improvement as a major health service objective. In order to monitor adherence to any policy which stresses the importance of improving clinical effectiveness, it is important that appropriate indicators of activity and outcomes are identified. Whilst such monitoring is not purely a central function, it would seem important that the NHS Management Executive is aware of the impact of one of its major policy initiatives.

Other potential national responsibilities for increasing the effectiveness of clinical interventions relate to both the provision and dissemination of relevant evidence. If reliable results are to be achieved, systematic reviews require considerable time and effort from people familiar with review methodology and skilled in critical appraisal of research evidence. Since such individuals are in short supply it is important that reviews are commissioned in a well co-ordinated manner so as to prevent duplication of effort. The NHS does have structures in place to achieve this, largely through its Research and Development Directorate. For example the constituent components of the Directorate's Information Systems Strategy (the UK Cochrane Centre, the NHS Centre for Reviews and Dissemination and the Project Register System) have a role in helping to co-ordinate review activity as do the regional directors of research and development and their networks. However, although structures are in place the precise mechanisms by which greater co-ordination is to be achieved have not yet been established and there continue to be examples of reviews being inappropriately commissioned with duplication of effort.

The NHS Research and Development Directorate has developed structures by which priorities can be identified that reflect the needs of both professionals in the NHS and consumers of its services. The prioritisation exercises undertaken so far have sought not just to identify topics for systematic review, but also for primary research. This is an important central role. Primary research into the effectiveness of clinical interventions should be directed to those areas where there is greatest uncertainty as well as significant potential for health service use before evidence of their cost effectiveness exists.

Systematic reviews must be made widely available if they are to have an impact in clinical practice. Marketing research draws a distinction between communications that merely increase awareness and those that may actually bring about changes of behaviour (Lomas 1993). In the latter there is more of an emphasis on personalised interactions, at a local rather than national level, in informal settings, with a message that incorporates local circumstances and which is ideally aimed at local opinion leaders.

Drawing on this model, Lomas has stressed the need for a credible dissemination body which synthesises and distributes research information. This would aim to raise awareness of research messages amongst professionals in general and support those individuals and organisations which may be able to bring about the implementation of the findings into clinical practice. The main responsibility of those bodies with a national remit would seem to be at the awareness-raising end of the dissemination spectrum, with implementation being the concern of organisations and individuals who work at a more local level.

There are a number of different organisations and agencies who already have or could legitimately develop such an awareness-raising role. They include the NHS Reviews and Dissemination Centre, the Department of Health, Health Care Directors and the Royal Colleges. It is important, however, that links between those who have a supra-district remit and those individuals and agencies who could have a direct role in local implementation are strengthened, and where necessary new networks formed. Although such a recommendation is not new, it would seem timely to re-emphasise the need so as to avoid the loss of results from the increasing activity in effectiveness research.

Local responsibilities

Given the requirements of a systematic review in terms of the resources and expertise required, there are probably only a few occasions when local healthcare purchasers and providers should undertake a review themselves. Both purchasers and providers of healthcare need to be aware of these areas where evidence of effectiveness exists and which can be used to guide local practice. For those topics where such evidence is missing, local agencies should make their needs known to the major research commissioners.

Implementing the results of research into clinical practice mostly requires local initiatives and mechanisms to be developed Grimshaw & Russell 1993b; Lomas 1993). Evidence of clinical effectiveness, either in the form of a systematic review or as part of nationally developed guidelines, often has to be adapted to local circumstances prior to its being successfully adopted and implemented. Although it would seem reasonable to assume that local individuals and organisations are best suited to this process, research discussed earlier in the chapter is inconclusive as to the extent that this should involve the end users. The actual implementation methods used will vary according to the behaviour which is to be changed. For instance, guidelines and decision support systems may be particularly useful in trying to influence individual clinical decisions about diagnosis and treatment.

If it were desired to prevent the use of an inappropriate surgical procedure, the commissioning process might be an effective lever in that commissioners could exclude such procedures from contracts. The promotion of a new surgical procedure may necessitate training of surgeons and, in some cases, provision of new equipment. Changing the organisation of care, for example to set up a stroke unit, is likely to be a more complex process involving administrative, organisational and potential change in skill mix of teams, which may encounter inertia and even opposition within institutions. There are important aspects of efficiency to be considered in this context, as Bentley *et al.* explain in Chapter 7.

Commissioners may have a significant role to play, for instance in developing and applying service specifications for specific clinical conditions in contracts. They can request providers to give evidence of the cost effectiveness of planned new developments in organisation of the service and in clinical practice. They also need to give consideration of how to overcome perverse incentives such as financial rewards for increased activity which may include ineffective care.

Increasingly, commissioners will be concerned with setting the parameters for clinical audit programmes and are therefore well placed to ensure that clinical effectiveness in specific fields is monitored. Despite the volume of audited activity, it is still difficult to get reliable information about the degree to which procedures of well proven effectiveness are being used. All too often it is necessary to mount potentially expensive one-off exercises to capture the appropriate data.

Commissioners may play a useful role in ensuring that routine data systems are improved. For instance, mother and child health data systems could be more closely tailored to monitoring the uptake of interventions evaluated in the Cochrane database.

Collaboration database: effective care in pregnancy and childbirth

Providers clearly have a central role to play in implementing research-based practice. Medical and clinical directors are likely to be increasingly involved in promoting clinical effectiveness and in some cases specific individuals are being identified in Trusts with a particular remit for R&D in general, and implementation in particular. Such individuals might function as change agents or opinion leaders with their colleagues.

Continuing professional development is an important means of promoting clinical effectiveness. Until now there have been few systematic attempts to link research output with educational programmes. Increasingly, it should be possible to develop educational materials based on systematic reviews and other rigorous sources of research-based information. In addition, professional education programmes are beginning to include teaching of critical appraisal skills and the application of information about diagnosis and treatment into individual clinical decisions. The growing awareness that professional development must be lifelong should be conducive to the wider dissemination of the skills needed to keep clinical performance up to date. The greatest change is likely to come when education, clinical audit and R&D are linked more closely. In the past these have been separate cultures and have often attracted different individuals. It now seems logical to bring them into a close working relationship. Miles *et al.*, writing in Chapters 3 and 4, specifically consider both the theoretical and operational mechanisms through which integration of clinical audit, R&D and general quality assurance may take place within provider organisations. They additionally consider how continuing medical education may be functionally linked to clinical audit as a central mechanism in achieving clinical guideline implementation into routine practice.

Users of the health service, either as members of groups or as individuals, could have an increasingly important role to play in clinical effectiveness. In the UK the National Childbirth Trust uses *Effective Care in Pregnancy and Childbirth* in training its own staff (Stocking 1993). Increasingly it is making research-based information available to its members. In the US, the Agency for Health Care Policy and Research has given wide publicity to its programme to develop guidelines on a range of topics. In Switzerland a successful campaign to reduce high rates of hysterectomy involved publicity in newspapers, radio and television (Domenighetti *et al.* 1988). Interactive videodiscs are now being developed on a range of topics, including prostatic hypertrophy, the treatment of breast cancer and hormone replacement therapy, in order to provide research-based evidence to patients about the outcomes of treatment in a way which allows them to participate more fully in the decision-making process. Such materials are currently under evaluation (Kasper *et al.* 1992). The advent of new technologies, such as video on demand, may further enhance the possibilities for sharing such information with patients. This is of central concern to patient organisations, as Rigge explains in Chapter 11.

Promoting clinical effectiveness – requirements for the future

An important consideration for any policy which aims to promote clinical effectiveness is whether the relevant skills exist to assist in the policy's success. In terms of the provision of information about clinical effectiveness, there is a lack of expertise in a number of relevant areas. The UK has relatively few individuals with the necessary health service research skills to support an extensive programme of primary research into the effectiveness of clinical interventions (Culyer 1994). There is also a relative lack of expertise in systematic reviews, not just in terms of carrying them out, but also in being able to appraise their quality. Many healthcare professionals are unaware that systematic reviews involve a formal methodology in keeping with other research methods. In some health authorities for example, registrars in public health medicine may be asked to undertake a review without appropriate training. In addition, they are often given only sufficient resources to review a small proportion of the relevant research, which in turn may have been identified in an ad hoc manner. If clinical effectiveness is to be improved in the UK, it would seem important that access to training programmes relevant to primary research methods, critical appraisal and systematic reviews should be increased. Ideally this should be carried out in a co-ordinated manner as part of a national strategy aimed not just at researchers, but also at clinicians and managers so they are better able to interpret research evidence appropriately.

Although a number of interventions have been shown to work in some circumstances, there remains considerable uncertainty about which to use in any particular set of conditions. In addition, some potential mechanisms such as NHS commissioning have not been evaluated adequately with respect to their potential to promote clinical effectiveness. This issue is examined in Chapter 8.

Decisions about which approaches to use in the implementation of a particular message should therefore reflect not just evidence from research but local knowledge and judgement. This may necessitate the development of training programmes to help develop these skills amongst healthcare professionals. Once particular interventions have been identified as having the potential to implement a particular research message, their resource implications should be considered before a final decision on their application is made. This process should involve not just consideration of the financial implications, but other factors such as the skills required by the intervention. Alternatively there are a number of groups, such as medical and pharmaceutical advisors in Family Health Service Authorities and public health practitioners, who could potentially take on such a role as an extension of their present duties. However, it is unclear whether these groups would agree to such a development, but if the approach is found to be cost effective potential detailers will require training in the technique.

The use of opinion leaders is another approach that has potential value in implementation. In the UK, it remains unclear how best to identify opinion leaders within clinical care, or even whether some specialties, for example general practice, recognise the existence of such individuals at all. In addition, most reported projects which have used opinion leaders have used them directly to persuade their colleagues about the benefits of a suggested approach to practice, rather in the manner of a 'detailer'. It is uncertain whether this technique would be acceptable to UK physicians, given their historical reluctance to intrude into a colleague's practice.

Similar questions exist for many of the other implementation interventions. Many of the most promising evaluations of audit and feedback as tools to promote clinical effectiveness involve the feedback being given in an individualised manner by a person in a position of authority. This is mostly counter to the way in which clinical audit is currently undertaken in the NHS and once again it is not clear whether such an approach would be possible in the UK. The use of reminder systems, though shown to be effective in some circumstances, also has implications for the NHS. Their design, particularly of computerised decision support systems, requires expertise and the extent to which this exists in the NHS is unclear, although this could be overcome by using outside contractors to do the design work. Ideally this should be centrally co-ordinated, although the wide variation in computer systems across the NHS would mitigate against this. The impact of such systems must also be formally evaluated.

Whichever approaches are used to disseminate research evidence and promote clinical effectiveness, costs will be incurred. Few studies to date, particularly in the UK, have provided cost data by which to compare the cost effectiveness of the possible approaches. Such considerations are particularly important for individual commissioning authorities which have a limited budget to purchase healthcare. If they are to optimise the health gain they can achieve for their local population, the benefits obtained from promoting clinical effectiveness should be greater than the costs incurred in disseminating the evidence and monitoring its uptake. It is therefore apparent that decisions about which approaches to use in the dissemination of evidence of effectiveness should be informed by a number of factors. For example, the skills required to undertake particular implementation methods; the cultural and professional norms of target professional groups; and the likely ratio of costs to benefits. Whilst dissemination needs to be guided by research evidence, methods used in the context of a research study cannot be translated wholesale into the NHS on the assumption that they will be successful without reference to other factors.

Future research priorities and conclusion

A policy to improve clinical effectiveness should ideally define future research needs. At present there are relatively few areas for which clear and reliable evidence of cost effectiveness exists. There continues to be a need, therefore, for both primary research and systematic reviews to be undertaken in order to identify the effectiveness and cost effectiveness of clinical interventions in use. In addition, the new technologies being developed should have an assessment of their effectiveness made before they are introduced into mainstream practice. Such a research plan also needs to be supported by a programme which seeks to develop further the methods of primary research and systematic review. This is a massive agenda and should be undertaken according to priorities which reflect the needs of the NHS and consumers of its services. The NHS R&D programme has set up and continues to develop structures which can address these issues. However, the challenges highlighted are relevant to healthcare systems throughout the world and, ideally, there should be strategies for international collaboration as well as national coordination. One of the most exciting ventures in this respect is the Cochrane Collaboration which is an international network of individuals and institutions committed to preparing, maintaining and disseminating systematic reviews.

Further research is needed to help clarify the dissemination of evidence on effectiveness. Both qualitative and quantitative research is necessary in order that knowledge is increased, not just of effective mechanisms by which research evidence can be incorporated into practice, but also of the context in which such mechanisms should be applied. A programme of evaluation of potential implementation strategies was commissioned in 1995 as part of the NHS R&D programme.

The recently established Cochrane Collaboration on Effective Professional Practice (CCEPP) will aid this process by providing overviews of the relevant and reliable research to date. A national research programme on methods of implementation will commission research on a range of interventions to promote clinical effectiveness and on factors which may influence the uptake of research findings so that in a few years much more will be known about effective implementation strategies in the NHS.

References

Anonymous (1992) Feasibility, safety and efficacy of domiciliary thrombolysis by general practitioners: Grampian region early anistreplase trial. *British Medical Journal* **305**: 548–53.

Antman, E., Lau, J., Kupelnick, B., Mosteller, F. & Chalmers, I. (1992) A comparison of the results of meta-analysis of randomized controlled trials and recommendations of clinical experts. *Journal of the American Medical Association* **268**: 240–48.

Birkhead, J.S. (1992) Time delays in provision of thrombolytic treatment in six hospitals. *British Medical Journal* **305**: 445–8.

Bobbio, M., Demichelis, B. & Giustetto G. (1994) Completeness of reporting trial results: effects on physicians' willingness to prescribe. *Lancet* **343**: 1209–11.

Chalmers, I., Dickersin, K. & Chalmers, T.C. (1992) Getting to grips with Archie Cochrane's Agenda. *British Medical Journal* **305**: 786–8.

Cluzeau, F., Littlejohns, P. & Grimshaw, J.M. (1994) Appraising clinical guidelines: towards a 'Which' guide for purchasers. *Quality in Health Care* **3**: 121–2.

Cochrane, A.L. (1972) *Effectiveness and Efficiency. Random Reflections on Health Services*, Nuffield Provincial Hospitals Trust, London.

Cochrane Collaboration (1993) *Effective Care in Pregnancy and Childbirth* database, (Cochrane updates available on disc), Oxford Update Software, Oxford.

Coulter, A., Klassen, A., Mackenzie, I.Z. & McPherson K. (1993) Diagnostic dilatation and curettage, is it used appropriately? *British Medical Journal* **306**: 236–9.

Culyer, D.A. (1994) *Supporting Research and Development in the NHS*, HMSO, London.

Davis, D.A., Thomson, M.A., Oxman, A.D. & Haynes, B. (1992) Evidence for the effectiveness of CME. *Journal of the American Medical Association* **268**: 1111–17.

Domenighetti, G., Luraschi, P., Gutzwiller, F., Pedrinis, E., Casabianca, A. & Spinelli, A. (1988) Effective information campaign by the mass media on hysterectomy rates. *Lancet* **ii**: 1470–73.

Donaldson, L. (1992) Maintaining excellence. *British Medical Journal* **288**: 903–905.

Eager, M. & Davey-Smith, G. (1995) Misleading meta-analysis. *British Medical Journal* **310**: 752–4.

Fendrick, A.M., Escarce, J.J., McLane, C., Thea, J.A. & Schwartz, J.S. (1994) Hospital adoption of laparoscopic cholecystectomy. *Medical Care* **32**: 1038–63.

Fibrinolytic Therapy Trialists Group (1994) Indications for fibrinolytic therapy in suspected acute myocardial infarction: collaborative overview of early mortality and major morbidity results from all randomised trials of more than 1000 patients. *Lancet* **343**: 11–22.

Freemantle, N., Grilli, R., Grimshaw, J.M., Russell, I. & Eccles, M. (1995) Implementing the findings of medicine. The Cochrane Collaboration on Effective Professional Practice. *Quality in Health Care* **4**: 45–7.

Goldberg, H.I., Cummings, M.A., Steinberg, E.P., Ricci, E.M., Shannon, T. & Soumerai, S.B. (1994) Deliberations of the dissemination of PORT products: translating research findings into improved patients outcomes. *Medical Care* **32** (Suppl.): JS90–JS110.

Grimes, D.A. (1993) Technology follies. *Journal of the American Medical Association* **342**: 31–50.

Grimshaw, J.M. & Russell, I.T. (1993a) Effects of clinical guidelines on medical practice: a systematic review of rigorous evaluations. *Lancet* **342** 1317–22.

Grimshaw, J.M. & Russell, I.T. (1993b) Achieving health gain through clinical guidelines I: Developing scientifically valid guidelines. *Quality in Health Care* **2**: 243–8.

Guyatt, G., Cook, D.J. & Jaeschke, R. (1995) How should clinicians use the results of randomized trials? *ACP Journal Club* January/February A12–13.

Haines, A., & Jones, R. (1994) Implementing the findings of research. *British Medical Journal* **308**: 1488–92.

Johnson, M.E., Langton, K.B., Haynes, R.B. & Mathieu, A. (1994) Effects of computer-based clinical decision support systems on clinician performance and patient outcome. A critical appraisal of research. *Annals of Internal Medicine* **120**: 135–42.

Kasper, J., Mulley, A. & Wennberg, J. (1992) Developing shared decision making programs to improve the quality of health care. *Quality Review Bulletin* **18**: 182–90.

Lomas, J. (1993) *Teaching Old (and not so old) Docs New Tricks: effective ways to implement research findings*, Centre for Health Economics and Policy Analysis, McMaster University, Hamilton, Ontario.

Mulrow, C.D. (1987) The medical review article; state of the science, *Annals of Internal Medicine* **104**: 470–71.

Mulrow, C.D. (1994) Rationale for systematic reviews. *British Medical Journal* **309**: 597–9.

NHSME (1993) *Improving Clinical Guidelines*, EL(93)115, NHS Management Executive, Department of Health, Leeds.

NHSME (1994) *Improving the Effectiveness of the NHS*, EL(94)74, NHS Management Executive, Department of Health, Leeds.

Nuffield Institute for Health (1994) *Effective Health Care. Implementing Clinical Guidelines*, Bulletin No. 8, University of Leeds, Leeds.

Oxman, A.D. (1994) Checklist for review articles. *British Medical Journal* **309**: 648–51.

Oxman A. In press Canadian Med. Assoc. J 1995.

Patterson-Brown, L.S., Wyatt, J.C. & Fisk, N.M. (1993) Are clinicians interested in up to date reviews of effective care? *British Medical Journal* **307**: 1464.

Pollitt, C., Hanson, S., Hunter, D.J. & Marnoch, G. (1992) General Management in the NHS: the initial impact. *Public Administration* **1**: 61–83.

Putnam, R.W. & Curry, L. (1985) Impact of patient care appraisal on physician behaviour in the office setting. *Canadian Medical Association Journal* **132**: 1025–9.

Putnam, R.W. & Curry, L. (1989) Physicians' participation in establishing criteria for hypertension management in the office: will patient outcomes be improved? *Canadian Medical Association Journal* **140**: 806–9.

Rogers, E.M. (1983) *Diffusion of Innovations.* Free Press, New York.

Sommers, L.S., Sholtz, R. & Shepherd, R.M. (1984) Physician involvement in quality assurance. *Medical Care* **22**: 1115–38.

Stocking, B. (1993) Implementing the findings of *Effective Care in Pregnancy and Childbirth. Milbank Quarterly* **71**: 497–522.

Thompson, S.G. (1994) Why sources of heterogeneity in meta-analysis should be investigated. *British Medical Journal* **309**: 1351–5.

Van Amringe, M. & Shannon, T.E. (1992) Awareness, assimilation and adoption: the challenge of effective dissemination and the first AHCPR-sponsored guidelines. *Quality Review Bulletin* **18**: 397–404.

6 ◆ Increasing the Appropriateness of Clinical Practice

Declan F. O'Neill

Introduction

Western healthcare delivery in the latter half of the twentieth century has been characterised by moves to adopt business management practices. The application of these practices is not confined to the management of healthcare organisations but is also relevant to clinical care, with varying degrees of success. Health carers have become members of teams which operate in markets selling their services to purchasers. Some carers are also purchasing care or influencing purchasing on behalf of their patients. Clinical services themselves have become organised into departments or directorates setting budgets, producing business plans, practising quality improvement, negotiating service contracts and having board level representation within their organisation. The concepts of clinical appropriateness and utilisation review have grown out of these philosophies and are considered here.

Industrial principles in healthcare management

The application of service industry management principles to healthcare can be beneficial in providing a different perspective to the processes involved in the delivery of clinical care, particularly through the introduction of methodologies for assuring quality and monitoring efficiency and effectiveness. The attendant risk lies in the over-zealous application of management principles to processes, the complexity of which is not fully understood.

Part of the difficulty encountered in applying these management principles to clinical care systems is that they do not easily fit. Clinical care delivery viewed in this manner would see the clinician in the role of product designer (the products being items of healthcare). Unlike the situation in most other industries, the clinician also manages production, and the range of products can be as broad as the number of patients treated. There are, however, certain advantages to be gained from using this perspective. In 'managing production' the clinician is dependent on a highly skilled team. The make up of the team may not be stable, in fact the components of all the support that a clinician may need to use could, theoretically, vary to the same degree as the range of 'products' being produced. In addition, some of that support may come from outside the clinicians' own department or practice.

In the clinical setting, defining or even perceiving the extent of that support and the complexities of its interconnections may be difficult. The clinician relies considerably on short term clinical outcomes and results to monitor the performance of the support. Much of this monitoring is done by intuition rather than by direct review and in practice would be confined to the noting of exceptions to the routine performance.

In general, clinical audit concentrates on specific clinical issues or areas of clinical priority and tends to focus on issues which are relatively overt. There are, however, many processes within the complex system of clinical care delivery where opportunities for maintaining or improving quality of service delivery may not make themselves apparent at all to the clinician. For example, a patient presents with a clinical picture for which clinical management indicates the taking of a biopsy of a particular organ or area of the body. The biopsy in question is then subjected to numerous tests by the histopathology service in order to investigate the possibility of various disease processes. These tests which are routine for the histopathology department require, say, four days, and the department is not in a position to provide a report until all testing is complete. If the clinical picture in question is rare it may well be that the clinician rarely has occasion to order such an investigation and is not at all aware of the time lapse between ordering the test and receiving the results. When further management options are dependent on the biopsy result there may be no further investigations or treatment carried out in the interim.

This scenario is not uncommon in a busy acute hospital unit where the in-patient is reviewed at the daily ward round and the conclusion of deliberations is 'awaiting results, review again tomorrow'. Because there is a mandatory four-day process to produce these particular results the same deliberation occurs on three days or, if a weekend intervenes, perhaps more. This example itself is concrete and may be a little extreme. There are, however, a myriad of subtle processes of a similar nature in the complex multiple network system of everyday clinical care in both the acute and community sectors, and in general practice. Of course they are by no means confined to the investigation processes and will include all manner of support systems and referral networks.

Because of the nature of the processes and the speed at which things change, because of the culture of clinical practice and the sheer volume of complex interrelations and processes involved, it may be unrealistic to expect any clinician to be intuitively in control of the sum of the effects of these factors on the efficient delivery of clinical care. Finding ways to evaluate these factors and to control their effects has occupied clinicians and researchers for some time. Some of the techniques emerging are being applied to the management of clinical services.

Managing utilisation

Examination of the utilisation of acute services must consider two aspects, overutilisation and underutilisation.

Overutilisation can occur from poor scheduling of services through earlier than necessary in-patient admission, through delays in the discharge process after a patient is fit to leave hospital or because of operational delays during an in-patient stay which result in hospital days that provide no benefit to the patient. It can be the result of an in-patient being placed in an acute unit when an alternative level of care would have been appropriate. It can also result from overservicing. It is not that uncommon, for example, for an investigation to be repeated when the results of a previous investigation are lost to the system, or perhaps for an investigation to be performed without due consideration of the expected additional information to be gained as a result. Similarly, as evidence on what is effective care accumulates, it is becoming apparent that there may be substantial numbers of procedures performed unnecessarily.

The undesirable effects of overutilisation are obvious. In terms of quality, there are the unnecessary risk of iatrogenic illness related to procedures, investigations or medications and the risk of hospital acquired infections. In terms of economics there is the wastage of scarce resources which could be more efficiently used otherwise.

Under-utilisation can occur in a number of ways. The first is the failure to identify a need for care. This falls outside the direct scope of utilisation management and review but is nevertheless relevant. As techniques for needs assessment improve, more demand for healthcare will be likely to arise, increasing the urgency for attention to efficiency and effectiveness. As over-utilisation may be the result of patients being inappropriately placed at a higher than necessary level of care, the corollary can be a cause of under-utilisation. Blocked beds can result in queues of appropriate cases unable to receive timely treatment. Under-utilisation may also occur if patients are discharged too early. In terms of quality, under-utilisation can lead to decreased functional status and quality of life, relapse, readmission and mortality. From an economic point of view, under-utilisation through delayed care, poor outcomes and cost to the individual and society, has a negative effect.

Utilisation management is described as action by clinicians, hospital management or purchasers to increase the efficiency and effectiveness of acute clinical care. What are the ways in which the delivery of care can be affected? The first task is to look at the delivery of care and look at what barriers may exist that prevent optimal clinical care delivery. This was described by Restuccia and Holloway (1976) in their seminal work on the subject. A 'barrier' to appropriate utilisation is the reason for a patient remaining in the acute hospital despite the determination that he could be appropriately cared for at an alternative level of care. The barriers to appropriate utilisation fall into four major groups according to responsibility:

- clinician responsibility
- hospital responsibility
- patient or family responsibility
- environmental responsibility.

Lists of the individual barriers (reasons for inappropriate use) can then be identified and classified according to cause type such as in the following examples:

- decision to discharge delayed
- organisation problem for scheduling procedure
- no family support
- social admission because alternative facilities not available.

A few common barriers were found to be responsible for the majority of misutilisation episodes. Since these were first described, much work has been done on the evaluation of misutilised hospital bed days and on ways of dealing with them. The following section will deal with evaluation methods in detail.

On the assumption that such barriers are identifiable it follows that good management, both at departmental level, and at organisation level, would wish to take steps to reduce or remove them. The goal of such internal management action is to influence the scheduling, location and process of providing care. The wider goals of clinical and purchaser strategies may involve modifying the external environment to provide alternative types and levels of care. Utilisation management therefore looks, initially at least, at process rather than outcome. This might seem to run counter to contemporary health philosophy where needs and outcomes are given pride of place. However, it is essential that the easier question of clinical appropriateness in terms of efficient use be comprehensively addressed in the first place, to improve clinical and patient outcomes through the efforts that go into identifying need and developing effectiveness over the longer period.

Utilisation management complements quality management. Strategies aimed at effecting utilisation should be closely aligned with quality strategies. Clinical management needs the ability to monitor the effects of one against the other to ensure that they remain complementary. For example if a unit was demonstrated to be operating at maximum occupancy with negligible 'inappropriateness', any further increase in throughput would carry substantial risk of diminishing quality.

Utilisation review

Utilisation review is the review of a patient's care through application of defined criteria and expert opinion. This is usually done through medical record reviews but various other methods, such as patient or staff interviews, are also described.

Although many people in different parts of the world have

researched ways for evaluating care used, the major impetus for development in this area came from US government policy in response to rising healthcare costs. From the start of the 1960s, utilisation review in its earliest form was emerging on a voluntary basis in progressive hospitals. By 1965 some commitment to utilisation review was being required of Medicare-participating hospitals. In 1972 legislation was enacted in the form of amendments to that country's Social Security Act, which included the Professional Standards Review Organisation (PSRO) programme (DHEW 1974). Under this legislation, committees or groups of doctors called PSROs were established at all participating hospitals. Their role was to review institutional services with priority given to review of hospital care under certain government health programmes. Different types of review were proposed:

(1) Retrospective and concurrent review – This envisaged, over time, the development of sets of criteria against which in-patient admissions and subsequent days of stay could be checked. Batches of cases are initially screened by trained nurse reviewers. Those cases found not to have met any criteria at the initial screen would then be rechecked by a clinician reviewer and then, where further indicated, by a peer review committee. The two-phase approach was aimed at, first, assuring at admission review that a hospital level of care is medically necessary, and second, placing a length of stay checkpoint on certified admissions for continued stay review. Initially introduced as retrospective review of cases after the hospital stay this gave rise to controversy over 'retrospective denials of payments' and led to concurrent review of patients as they were being admitted. This process has evolved into what is commonly known as utilisation review.

(2) Medical care evaluation studies – This technique was envisaged as a method for emphasising quality improvement through continuing medical education. It proposed specifically to correct identified problems via a structured review process through medical audit pathways, education processes and repeated review. It represents what is now referred to as clinical audit.

(3) Profile analysis – This activity involves retrospective review of aggregated patient care data subjected to various pattern analyses, such as lengths of stay, resource usage and adjusted risk, according to casemix, clinician, specialty, hospital and so on.

Types of utilisation review

Different types of utilisation review are described. They fall into four main categories:

(1) Implicit criteria – A clinician reviewer directly applies his own judgement to quality and/or appropriateness of the care

provided. Validity depends entirely on knowledge, skill and judgement of the reviewer.

(2) Length of stay (LOS) profiles – The title is self explanatory. Casemix structured profiles are used. They are generally designed to reflect mean clinical LOS for region or district, mean peer LOS for unit or hospital, and to provide exception reporting for cases outside two standard deviations from the mean.

(3) Explicit criteria (diagnosis independent) – This is a level of care criteria audit. These instruments consist of standard sets of criteria which reflect the severity of illness and intensity of service which justifies admission. They include criteria which define levels of medical services, nursing services and patient conditions (not diagnosis specific) which require continuing acute hospital in-patient stay. They are used for screening activity through recorded patient information (the medical record) in conjunction with a review by clinicians of incidences where no criteria are met.

(4) Explicit criteria (diagnosis specific) – This is a diagnostic criteria audit. Individual guidelines are established for specific categories of patients and conditions. The guidelines are complex instruments whose establishment represents a substantial workload based on evidence and expert consensus relating to the appropriateness of the care provided for a particular set of clinical circumstances. The review process is structured and complex in itself.

Methods of use

All of these types of utilisation review instruments have been used at different stages in different environments.

Implicit criteria

When researchers first started to examine the utilisation of clinical services, the use of implicit criteria was common. In these studies the decision as to whether or not a referral, an attendance, an admission or a day of stay is appropriate is made by the reviewer. The validity of such methods depends entirely on the skills, judgement and knowledge of the reviewer (Donabedian 1982). The inherent weakness in this approach is the inconsistency found to exist between clinician reviewers. Agreement rates using these techniques have been described as being at or near the level expected by chance alone (Sanzaro 1980).

Methods for overcoming this weakness have included: stratification of cases into subgroups based on casemix, lengths of stay and other such parameters; the inclusion and weighting of a range of opinion groups such as patients, carers, general practitioners, nursing staff, junior doctors and consultants; the prior development of consensus opinion for a range of condition states through Delphi-type techniques, with incorporation into the decisions on appropriateness. All of these modifications were found to have their own cost. It has been common experience that the more the instruments are enhanced the more cumbersome they become to use.

This difficulty has led to the development (described below) of explicit criteria type instruments, however their use has been mainly confined, so far, to acute in-patient services or to specific conditions or procedures. In general, studies investigating referral pathways or the use of ambulatory care or non-acute care must still rely on this type of instrument.

Length of stay profiles

Of particular use for examining the margins of a tranche of clinical activity are 'length of stay profiles' and other similar techniques which focus on parameters directly related to patterns of service consumption. The aim with this type of exercise is to create utilisation profiles for specific areas of activity such as whole hospitals, specialty units, discrete wards or procedure units, or individual clinician workloads. The origins of such profiles were based on casemix and lengths of stay for different clinician groups, and there is no limit to the range of variables which can be used to create a profile of activity.

The profile is presented in terms of the distribution of overall activity. The cases falling outside (say) two standard deviations for a particular variable, e.g. length of stay, are then examined in further detail for underlying factors which may (or may not) be reducible or avoidable. The main limitation with this type of exercise is that it focuses on what is marginal; it provides little or no information about the bulk of activity. The technique can, however, be particularly useful for homing in on high cost, high risk, high dependency or other particular aspects of a clinical service.

Explicit criteria (diagnosis independent)

These instruments remain in common use and have been refined over the years. The use of two such instruments has been widespread in North America. They are the Appropriateness Evaluation Protocol (AEP) (Gertman & Restuccia 1981) and the Intensity, Severity, Discharge screens-A (ISD-A) (InterQual Inc. 1987). This type of utilisation review is relatively simple and inexpensive and is showing potential for effective application in the NHS environment, particularly at a local clinical management level.

The instruments have been shown to be quite sensitive in determining the levels of efficient utilisation of acute services. One such tool, the AEP and its paediatric modification PAEP have demonstrated sensitivities of 90% or over (Gertman & Restuccia 1981; Kempner 1988). However, when used in the PSRO programme some of the sensitivity and specificity of these instruments appears to be lost (Dippe *et al.* 1989).

It has been noted by the developers of the AEP that specific agreement rates for inappropriateness were higher if reviewers were familiar with the institution in question and its clinical capabilities (Restuccia 1982). A good case exists, therefore, for using these instruments directly within clinical audit rather than as a form of external review, such as that required by PSRO programme. Evidence of difficulties associated with remote use has already been noted in a UK experiment, (referred to in more detail below).

The instruments themselves consist of lists of criteria which reflect the need for care, severity and dependency, such as:

- intravenous medications and/or fluid replacement (excluding tube feedings)
- loss of ability to move a limb or other body part within 48 hours of admission (excluding trauma)
- Severe electrolyte/acid-base abnormality
- ECG evidence of acute ischaemia with suspicion of new MI.

(Abbreviated and adapted from Restuccia (1986). The instruments may be arranged in functional groups such as patient condition and clinical services, as in the AEP, or into intensity, severity and discharge groups or into other logical groupings, as in the ISD-A.

As the distribution of barriers to appropriate utilisation is known to change after admission (Restuccia & Holloway 1976), different criteria lists are used for evaluation of admission days and days of stay. For example, the AEP instrument contains 16 admission day criteria and 25 days of stay criteria.

In the standard method of use the instruments are applied by screening in-patient medical records against the criteria. If any one of the criteria is met the admission or subsequent day of stay is considered appropriate. Those records where no criteria were met are then subjected to a further review by a panel of clinicians. This phase of the process is designed to incorporate clinical expertise in order to identify appropriate care not encompassed by the criteria. Where a case is considered appropriate although not having met any criteria, the reviewing clinicians operate an override to include it with those deemed appropriate. For the remaining cases reasons for inappropriateness are ascertained and recorded. The result of a survey provides an estimate of appropriate utilisation and a profile of the underlying reasons for inappropriate utilisation. Different modes of use are described:

(1) Retrospective, where a sample of in-patients' records from a period in the recent past are examined. Any conclusions drawn from the findings are applied to current management practice in order to demonstrate change at future review.

(2) Concurrent, where review is conducted on the records of current in-patients. As barriers to appropriateness are recognised the information is fed back to the responsible clinicians to stimulate change 'concurrently'.

(3) Prospective, where instead of reviewing the status of the patient on or after admission, the criteria are used for admission and confirmed stay policy guidelines that consider the appropriateness or otherwise of an admission, prior to the patient arriving in hospital or the appropriateness of continued stay after a stated period.

An example of the type of reasons for inappropriate use and the progress made towards modifying them is shown in Figures 6.1 and 6.2. These results are from two surveys of the same hospital, taken 18 months apart. The first survey found 17.6% inappropriate admission days and 17.8% inappropriate days of stay. In the second survey, these were found to have dropped to 8.7% and 9.2% respectively (O'Neill *et al.* 1992).

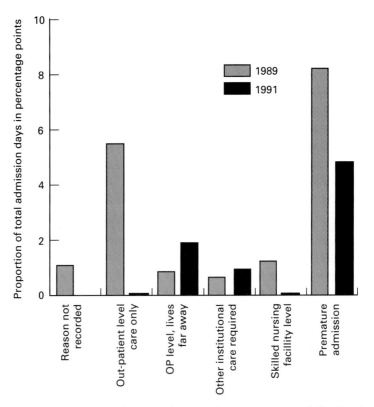

Fig. 6.1   Inappropriate admission days – primary reasons and distribution.

Explicit criteria (diagnosis specific)
The fourth type of review instrument has been developed through the incorporation of evidence and consensus based clinical guidelines into criteria sets. These criteria sets outline the specific circumstances where the use of a particular clinical procedure or line of clinical management is clearly appropriate, those where it is of doubtful appropriateness,

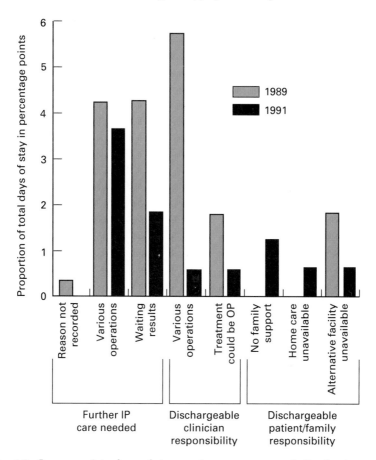

Fig. 6.2   Inappropriate days of stay – primary reasons and distribution.

and those where it is clearly inappropriate. These can be applied through computer algorithms which are then used to review the indications for admission and continued care.

The uses and benefits of clinical guidelines are dealt with in detail in various places throughout this volume. The approach to guideline development and implementation varies both between and within countries. In the UK much of the activity in clinical guideline development has taken place at local level, in and between primary and secondary care and in conjunction with commissioners. The common vehicle which has the potential to draw these agents together in a co-ordinated approach on shared priorities is clinical audit. The practice of clinical audit is a contractual requirement of doctors employed in the NHS. Such audit is also an increasingly common component of contract specifications for clinical services. Commissioner tutelage is further strengthened by the requirement for a proportion (40%) of the clinical audit agenda to address purchaser priorities (NHSME 1994). This is supported at national level by a number of initiatives and one of these is the work of a subcommittee of the Chief Medical Officer for

England's Clinical Outcomes Group which has commissioned pilot projects on national guidelines. Other initiatives include the work of the Cochrane Centre in Oxford and its participation in the wider Cochrane Collaboration, the Centre for Dissemination of Reviews at the University of York, the Outcomes Clearing House at the Nuffield Institute in Leeds, the production of the effectiveness bulletins, the work of the Central Outcomes Unit of the Department of Health in England and that of the Clinical Outcomes project of the Welsh Office.

In the USA, Holland, France and elsewhere, substantial effort has gone into the development of national clinical guidelines for ever enlarging lists of clinical practice areas along with ways of encouraging their implementation. This trend may in part reflect the type of healthcare systems operating in particular countries. The use of methods which encourage adherence to clinical guidelines, particularly in health insurance reimbursement based systems is seen, by some, as a way of improving both the efficiency and the quality of the services purchased. In the USA the Health Care Financing Administration has directly funded the national guideline development programme. Much of the related work has been conducted by RAND Corporation and the University of California. The RAND/UCLA approach seeks to create the means for deciding whether a particular clinical practice is appropriate. The definition of appropriateness used by RAND/UCLA is:

'Appropriate that the expected health benefit exceeds the expected negative consequences by a sufficiently wide margin that the procedure is worth doing'

(Brook 1991).

Methods which incorporate consensus-derived guidelines into explicit criteria diagnosis-specific utilisation review instruments have been described in detail (Chassin 1989). In summary they consist of a number of steps which start with a literature review of the known evidence on the efficacy and effectiveness of a particular practice. This is followed by the creation of long lists of possible indications for the practice, the development of patient classes based on symptomatology and groups of clinical signs and the identification of critical clinical decision making factors for each group. A panel of expert clinicians is identified (with those who actually perform the procedure or management method being in a minority). The panel members rate each of the indications in the list on a scale, with the top end of the scale being the maximum expression of benefits outweighing risk and the bottom end being the maximum expression of risks outweighing benefits. Through consensus development technique the ratings are refined into an agreed statement. The result of such an exercise is a list of appropriate, equivocal and inappropriate indications for a particular procedure, investigation or management programme. It then becomes possible to incorporate these into checklists or computer algorithms, thereby providing expert systems for clinical audit, decision analysis, utilisation review and managed care. These instruments are very specific, and they require significant resources to develop and to enable regular updating.

Experience and developments in utilisation management and review

United States of America

Utilisation management and review is widely practised in the USA. The driving philosophy behind its inception was to reduce the costs involved in acute care provision. With the diagnosis-independent instruments there have been attempts to shift to concurrent review in response to reported increased behaviour modification with this mode, as compared with the retrospective mode (Restuccia 1982). However, the practicalities of using them in this mode do not sit well with the type of reviews required of peer review organisation programmes.

Recent developments have seen increasing use of diagnosis-specific instruments. This means that the utilisation management brief has been widened, moving from a simple efficiency focus to include effectiveness. Certain insurers and health maintenance organisations have introduced proactive management of admissions and continued stay. Using computer-based checklists, selected admissions are screened for appropriateness. The application of computer-based diagnosis-independent instruments as a means of developing managed care is also described elsewhere (UMA 1993).

United Kingdom

In the UK, studies into the appropriateness of acute hospital use have been reported intermittently for over 30 years.

Implicit criteria instruments

A cluster of studies appeared towards the end of the 1950s. The first, consisting of medical record reviews and interviews with relatives of patients discharged from a Birmingham hospital, reported 'no diagnostic or therapeutic requirements at hospital level in a quarter of patients' (Crombie & Cross 1959). A second using consultant opinions reported similar findings for existing inpatients (Forsyth & Logan 1960). A further larger survey in Birmingham, this time on admissions and delayed discharges, reported 4.7% admissions and a further 13.3% of delayed discharges unnecessary on medical grounds alone (Mackintosh *et al.* 1961).

All of these studies used implicit clinical opinion in determining the appropriateness or otherwise of a case. Later, researchers used different ways to try to overcome the inherent weakness of implicit criteria: Torrance *et al.* (1972) channelled opinion into general categories of reasons for admission (e.g. consultant opinion required, alternative services unavailable) and introduced basic explicit needs criteria (medical needs, nursing needs, etc.); and Rosser (1976) put forward a method for incorporating consensus clinician opinion derived through local use of Delphi techniques. As elsewhere, these were found to be of doubtful validity across different environments or too cumbersome for practical wider use when heavily structured. They have continued to be reported for specific settings from time to time (Murphy 1977; Farag & Tinker 1985; Coid & Crome 1986; Beech *et al.* 1987).

Explicit criteria (diagnosis-independent) instruments
In 1972 a study which used a comprehensive explicit criteria instrument was reported in Northern Ireland (Donaldson *et. al.* 1972). This was roughly at the same time that the first explicit criteria instruments were appearing in the USA. This instrument comprised a set of criteria designed in conjunction with medical and nursing staff. The survey consisted of a screening of medical records followed by concurrent review on the wards with consultants. As there was no real groundswell for studying utilisation in the UK at the time, it seems that the research was not expanded upon.

In 1987, Anderson *et al.* reported the development of an audit instrument consisting of nine explicit criteria applied, through interviews with nursing staff, to in-patient days of stay, which they called the bed study instrument. The authors acknowledged similarity between their instrument and the AEP. The similarity can be found in the subject area of the majority of criteria, although the number of criteria and level of detail are less in the bed study instrument.

A recent study in Bristol at one acute site using the ISD-A instrument and validating against the AEP has reported a potential for altering patterns of care through use of lower intensity/dependency services in the region of 10–15% for general medicine and geriatrics and for reducing the length of stay of other admissions (Coast *et al.* 1994). The Royal College of Physicians administered a postal survey of medical admissions at 40 randomly chosen acute hospitals in which the instrument used was the AEP. Difficulties were reported in controlling for the clinical review element with the remote administration which was reflected in unacceptably high override rates in the clinical review phase (Houghton 1994). Further use of the bed study instrument (Victor *et al.* 1993; Victor & Khahoo 1994) on inner city hospitals has reported high appropriateness levels contrasting with those found in a provincial teaching hospital eight years earlier, various possible causes are cited.

In the recent past there have frequently been sporadic reports of hospitals experiencing increases in the proportion of emergency admissions (Hobbs 1995). This has given rise to an increasing interest in utilisation review. Single retrospective surveys with AEP have been conducted across four centres in north west Thames. 'Snapshot surveys' with a paediatric AEP at Great Ormond Street Children's Hospital and a modified bed study instrument in Rugby (Wernicke 1995, personal communication) are reported. A survey of 186 acute hospital emergency admissions using AEP in Buckinghamshire found high clinician override rates and suggested the need for extra criteria

(Lawrence and Edwards 1995). A survey of emergency medical admissions at Aintree, Liverpool using the AEP is reported (Bogg *et al* 1995). Use of the AEP for the specific purpose of identifying acute hospital bed usage which could be appropriately substituted with hotel beds is described (Harvey *et al* 1993).

Further prospective research into the validity and acceptance of this sort of evaluation of care is now being undertaken through some larger studies. A multi-centre three phase study using the adult AEP (locally modified) and cross validation studies with other instruments has commenced in south Thames (Beech *et al* 1995). Another multi-centre study is being established by the British Paediatric Association in Yorkshire using a paediatric version of the AEP (Smith 1995). A two site study using the bed study instrument and comparing with the AEP to monitor and evaluate the effect of a utilisation management strategy is in progress in East Kent (Fenn *et al* 1995).

Explicit criteria (diagnosis-specific) instruments
The use of diagnosis-specific instruments in the UK has been limited. Development of instruments on the lines described above took place in Trent region in the late 1980s (Hampton 1989). Currently a project has been established at Lewisham in south Thames in which diagnosis-specific instruments for upper GI endoscopy, tonsillectomy, grommets, dilatation and curettage, and hysterectomy are being modified and tested. The panels for the modification exercises are made up of two general practitioners, one internal specialist in the field from the hospital and one external specialist from elsewhere, a specialist clinician from an unassociated clinical specialty and a public health physician (Stott 1995).

Australia
Explicit criteria, diagnosis-independent tools have been piloted at a number of globally budgeted teaching hospital sites with levels of appropriateness of 80–95%+ being reported (O'Donnell *et al.* 1989, Oldham *et al.* 1991). Local adaptations of AEP instruments were used. Development of concurrent review for internal utilisation management has been described as has modification in utilisation in response to utilisation management (O'Neill *et al.* 1992).

Canada
A survey representative of Canadian acute care hospitals larger than 100 beds found 80% had a utilisation management programme (Anderson *et al.* 1990). The main reasons given for implementing utilisation management were high occupancy or funding issues rather than the direct cost containment incentive in the USA. In the USA there has traditionally been an over-abundant supply of acute care providers. Funding issues were particularly common in the Canadian province where funding had been connected to output (in terms of casemix utilisation).

Canadian hospitals are not profit making organisations and are funded through either global budgets or output based budgets. Anderson *et al.* pointed out the distinction between efficient and effective bed use on the one hand and cost control on the other. They noted that the former may give rise to a heavier casemix with resulting maintenance or increase of cost. Interestingly, the main approach to utilisation management in Canada at that stage had been through retrospective utilisation review using the explicit criteria, diagnosis-independent type instruments. The authors suggested that the lack of progression to the other modes of use could indicate either the ability to meet existing needs, or that utilisation management was in an early stage of evolution in Canada.

France
In France, interest in utilisation review has been growing in the field of medical audit. Most of the experience to date has been in emergency departments. A locally modified version of the AEP has been tested (Davido *et al* 1991). Reported studies describe the use of the instruments for evaluation of emergency department admissions (Duteil *et al.* 1994), applied prospectively using medical records and information acquired directly from patients (Lang 1995).

Ireland
Surveys of cohorts of longer stay patients in acute units are reported (Hynes *et al.* 1991).

Italy
A survey of studies conducted between 1988 and 1993 which looked at appropriateness, identified eleven utilisation review studies of varying types. Five of these studies were found to have data sufficiently comparable to be pooled. Modified versions of the AEP were used in all of the studies. Average levels of appropriateness were estimated from the pooled data as 77% of admissions and 58% of days of stay (Fellin *et al.* 1995).

Portugal
The Portuguese Ministry of Health has committed substantial investment to utilisation review since it funded research at four pilot sites in 1985. Utilisation review is currently conducted at all public hospitals using a nationally modified version of the AEP. National average levels of appropriateness are estimated to be running at 78% for admissions and 54% for subsequent days of stay (Benetes *et al.* l995).

Spain
A number of studies have been published with varied results (see O'Neill *et al.* (1996) for review). As in the UK, many more surveys have been conducted which are unpublished (Lorenzo 1994). With the

exception of the Gonzales-Montalvo study, utilisation review has been conducted retrospectively (Lorenzo & Sunol 1995).

Switzerland
A review of four studies at regional hospitals between 1989 and 1991 reported appropriateness levels of 84–92% for admissions and 94–98% for days of stay (Santos-Eggimann *et al.* 1995). One hospital is reported to have adopted routine utilisation review after conducting a pilot survey. The AEP and an instrument known as the delay tool (which provides further detail on the reasons for inappropriateness) are used. The process is part of the hospital's TQM/CQI programme and is used to develop predictive models (Blanc 1994). Explicit criteria diagnosis-specific instruments are being developed for local use in Lausanne using procedures similar to those chosen at Lewisham (Pacaud 1994).

Appropriateness of hospital use in Europe
A European study group has been established in 1994, through an EC Biomed project grant. Included in the group's objectives are the development of common core instruments for evaluating utilisation and the reasons underlying inappropriate utilisation (Liberati 1995).

Focused utilisation analysis and proactive management of utilisation

By conducting utilisation review, major barriers to appropriate utilisation become evident. Of those which fall within the responsibility of the organisation's internal management, some may be redressed through straightforward policy change or other management practice. For others – particularly subtle systematic practices or admissions – it may be desirable to introduce systematic clinical management processes to assist with their identification and with reorientation of practice. Recent NHS experience with two such practices is reported. Adverse Event Monitoring is the systematic detection, investigation and analysis of events which indicate or may indicate that a patient received poor quality care (Bennett & Walshe 1990).

Patient Focused Care is a detailed analysis system which looks at care from the patient's position, and uses a projection of the 'anticipated recovery pathway' for each type of patient. This enables the optimal pathways through the various care processes to be mapped. The mapping then reveals the common loci for barriers to good utilisation or factors detrimental to maintaining and improving quality (Bruce & Van Liew 1992).

Utilisation review and the healthcare system

The UK Department of Health has a stated policy position to move the focus of healthcare from the secondary/tertiary care sector to the primary care sector (DoH 1994). Shifting the focus includes shifting a certain amount of care. This position assumes that there is a significant caseload which is currently dealt with by the secondary/tertiary care sector and which could be more appropriately managed at an alternative level of care. Such a readjustment would then be expected to result in:

(1)   A decrease in the over-servicing of patients who are inappropriately receiving secondary level care.
(2)   A decrease in the under-servicing of patients who should appropriately be receiving primary and community level care.
(3)   Some potential to reduce the under-servicing of patients who should appropriately be receiving secondary level care but are either in the system but not receiving care or not being referred.

The difficulty in translating this theory into practice is in finding commonly agreed definitions of levels of care at any point in the system. Initial attention should be concentrated at the locus at which there is the strongest potential for influencing movement across levels. In the current situation many supposedly acute units find themselves responding to demands for services which may not be acute because there is no appropriate supply elsewhere. The need to define what is and what is not acute care is clear.

Systematic analysis of acute admission days and days of stay against an agreed set of criteria which indicate acute care can be used to assess a unit's activity. A study of the subgroups which fail to meet the criteria can be used to identify the major reasons why patients are receiving inappropriate care. Some of the reasons found will be amenable to internal managerial action. Other reasons will be identified which relate to barriers to appropriate use arising from the external environment. A further potential development is to devise criteria sets for other levels of care such as community hospitals, extended care units, hospital at home and services outside of the NHS such as nursing homes. For each of these situations it would be necessary to consider criteria which delineate more than one interface with other levels of care.

Conclusion

Studies of the appropriateness of clinical intervention and the practice of utilisation review are likely to play an increasingly important role in the management and rationalisation of modern healthcare. This chapter has aimed to describe the basic principles which underly these initiatives and to describe how they are being developed in the international setting. Properly managed, they show considerable potential in improving the quality of care delivered to patients.

References

Anderson, G., Sheps, S.B. & Cardiff (1990) Hospital based utilisation management, a cross-Canada survey. *Canadian Medical Association Journal* **143**: 1025–30.

Anderson, P., Meara, J., Broadhurst, S., Attwood, S., Timbrell, M. & Gatherer, A. (1987) Use of beds: a cohort study of admissions to a provincial teaching hospital. *British Medical Journal* **297**: 910–12.

Beech, R., Challah, S. & Ingram, R.S. (1987) Impact of cuts in acute beds on services for inpatients. *British Medical Journal* **29**: 685–8.

Beech, R., O'Neill, D.F. & Hesketh, T. (1995) *Analysing acute inpatient services in south Thames. The development and application of utilisation review tools. Preliminary report.* United Medical and Dental Schools Department of Public Health Medicine.

Benetes, M., Pina, E., Santos, M. & da Luz Gonsalves, D. (1995) *Utilisation review: the Portugese experience*, Prepared on behalf of the Appropriateness of Hospital Use in Europe Study Group, submitted for publication.

Bennett, J. & Walshe, K. (1990) Occurrence screening as a method of audit. *British Medical Journal* **300**: 1248–51.

Blanc, T. (1994) *State of Vaud public health department, Lausanne*, paper presented at the Appropriateness of Hospital Use in Europe workshop, Bergamo.

Bogg, J., Lee, A., Marie, F., Milne, K., O'Neill, C., Seddon, D., Thompson, C., Thurston, H. & Pearson, M. (1995) *Study of Emergency Medical Admissions at Aintree*, Health and Community Care Research Unit, University of Liverpool and North West RHA.

Brook, R.H. (1991) *Measures of Appropriateness, Quality Care and Health Status Available From RAND*, RAND, Santa Monica, CA.

Bruce, C. & Van Liew, J. (1992) *Integrated care*, paper presented to the British Association of Medical Managers Autumn Conference.

Chassin, M. (1989) How do we decide whether an investigation or procedure is appropriate? In: *Appropriate Investigation and Treatment in Clinical Practice* (ed. A. Hopkins), Royal College of Physicians of London, London, pp. 21–9.

Coast, J., Inglis, A., Morgan, K., Gray, S., Kanmerling, M. & Frankel, S. (1994) *The hospital admissions study: final report*, Health Care Evaluation Unit, University of Bristol.

Coid, J. & Crome, P. (1986) Bed blocking in Bromley. *British Medical Journal* **292**: 2153–6.

Crombie, D.L. & Cross, K.W. (1959) Implicit criteria instruments. *Medical Practice* **242**: 361–4.

Davido, A., Nicoulet, I., Levy, A. & Land, T. (1991) Appropriateness of admission in an emergency department: reliability of assessment and causes of failure. *Quality Assurance in Health Care* **3**: 227–34.

DHEW (1974) *PSRO Program Manual*, US Department of Health, Education and Welfare, Office of Professional Standards Review, US Government Printing Office, Washington, DC.

Dippe, S.E., Bell, M.M. & Wells, M. (1989) A peer review of peer-review organisations. *Western Journal of Medicine* **51**: 561.

DoH (1994) *Developing NHS Purchasing and GP Fundholding: Towards a Primary Care Led NHS*, EL(94) 79, Department of Health, London.

Donabedian, A. (1982) *Explorations in Quality Assessment and Monitoring. The Criteria and Standards of Quality*, vol II, Health Administration Press, Ann Arbor, MI.

Donaldson, S.N., Wheeler, M.R. & Barr, A. (1972) Demand for patient care. *British Medical Journal* **272**: 799–802.

Duteil, M., Le Chevalier, S., Le Coutour, X., Potier, J.C. & Bazin, C. (1994) Evaluation de la pertinence des hospitalisations demandées aux urgences medicales. *Reanimation Urgences* **2**: 111.

Farag, R.R. & Tinker, G.M. (1985) Delays in discharge of patients from an acute geriatric unit. *Health Trends* **17**: 44.

Fellin, G., Apolone, G., Tampieri, A., Bevilacqa, L., Mergalli, G., Minella, C. & Liberati, A. (1995) *Assessing the appropriateness of hospital use: an overview of the Italian experience*, Prepared on behalf of the Appropriateness of Hospital Use in Europe Study Group, submitted for publication.

Fenn, A., Horner, P., Travis, S., Prescott, G. & Bates, T. (1995) *Inappropriate bed usage in a district general hospital*, preliminary report, William Harvey Hospital and East Kent Health Authority.

Forsyth, G. & Logan, R.F.L. (1960) *The Demand for Medical Care*, Churchill Livingstone, London.

Gertman, P.M. & Restuccia, J.D. (1981) The Appropriateness Evaluation Protocol: a technique for assessing unnecessary days of hospital care. *Medical Care* **8**: 855–71.

Hampton, J.R. (1989) Appropriate use of investigations in cardiology. In: *Appropriate Investigation and Treatment in Clinical Practice*, (ed. A. Hopkins), Royal College of Physicians of London, London, pp. 31–9.

Harvey, J., Jenkins, R. & Llewellyn, L. (1993) Estimating the appropriateness of acute bed use: role of the patient hotel. *Journal of Epidemiology and Community Health.* **47**: 368–72.

Hobbs, R. (1995) Rising emergency admissions. *British Medical Journal* **310**: 207–208.

Houghton, A. (1994) *The Audit of Medical Admissions*, Royal College of Physicians, London.

Hynes, M., O'Herlihy, B.P., Laffoy, M. & Hayes, C. (1991) Patients 21 days or more in an acute hospital bed: appropriateness of care. *Irish Journal of Medical Science* **160**: 389–92.

InterQual Inc. (1987) *The ISD-A Review System with Adult Criteria. The ISD-A Review System with Paediatric Criteria*, Chicago, IL.

Kempner, K.J. (1988) Medically inappropriate hospital use in a paediatric population. *New England Journal of Medicine* **318**: 1033–7.

Lang, T. (1995) *Assessing the appropriateness of hospital use: an overview of the French experience*, Prepared on behalf of the Appropriateness of Hospital Use in Europe Study Group, submitted for publication.

Lawrence, D. & Edwards, G. (1995) *Emergency admissions and bed use*, Buckinghamshire Health Authority and FHSA, Milton Keynes General NHS Trust.

Liberati, A. (1995) *Appropriateness of hospital use: An EC Biomed European project assessing the medical appropriateness of hospital utilisation and its structural, financial and social determinants*, progress report, Mario Negri Institute, Milan.

Lorenzo, S. (1994) *Utilisation review*, paper presented at the Appropriateness of Hospital Use in Europe workshop, Bergamo.

Lorenzo, S. & Sunol, R. (1995) *Assessing the appropriateness of hospital use: an overview of the Spanish experience*, Prepared on behalf of the Appropriateness of Hospital Use in Europe Study Group, submitted for publication.

Mackintosh, J.M., McKeown, T. & Garrat, F.N. (1961) An examination of the need for hospital admission. *Lancet* **ii**: 815–18.

Murphy, F.W. (1977) Blocked beds. *British Medical Journal* **1**: 1395–6.

NHSME (1994) *Clinical audit: 1994/95 and beyond*, EL(94)20, National Health Service Management Executive, Department of Health, Leeds.

O'Donnell, J., Pilla, J., Van Gunert, L., Oldham, D. & Scuteri, J. (1989) *Evaluation of the Appropriateness of Hospital Admissions*, conference report, Royal Australian College of Medical Administrators, Melbourne.

Oldham, D., Scuteri, J. & O'Donnell, J. (1991) *Assessment of the Appropriateness of Utilisation Review Activities in Western Australian Hospitals,* Health Department of Western Australia/KPMG Peat Marwick Consultants.

O'Neill, D.F., Hicks, D. & Smalley, S. (1992) *Efficient use of acute inpatient services. Final report,* Fremantle Hospital, Kent.

O'Neill, D., Miles, A. & Polychronis, A. (1996) Central dimensions of clinical practice evaluation: efficiency, appropriateness and effectiveness I. *Journal of Evaluation in Clinical Practice* **2**: 13–27.

Pacaud, F. (1994) Personal communication to the author from Dr Fred Pacaud, Department of Public Health, University of Lausanne.

Restuccia, J.D. (1982) The effect of concurrent feedback in reducing inappropriate hospital utilisation. *Medical Care* **1**: 46–62.

Restuccia, J.D. (1986) The AEP User Manual.

Restuccia, J.D. & Holloway, D.C. (1976) Barriers to apppropriate utilisation of an acute facility. *Medical Care* **7**: 559–73.

Rosser, R.M. (1976) The reliability and application of clinical judgement in evaluating the use of hospital beds. *Medical Care* **XIVI**: 112–18.

Santos-Eggimann, B., Paccaud, F. & Blanc, T. (1995) *Medical appropriateness of hospital utilisation: an overview of Swiss studies,* Prepared on behalf of the Appropriateness of Hospital Use in Europe Study Group, submitted for publication.

Sanzaro, P.J. (1980) Quality assessment and quality assurance in medical care. *Annual Review of Public Health* **1**: 37–8.

Smith, H. (1995) Personal communication to be author from Dr Helen Smith, Wessex Primary Care Research Network.

Stott, R. (1995) Personal communication from to the author from Dr Robin Stott, Medical Director, Lewisham Hospital.

Torrance, N., Hogg, D. & Knox, J.D.E. (1972) Acute admissions to medical beds. *Journal of the Royal College of General Practitioners* **22**: 211–19.

UMA (1993) *Managed Care Appropriateness Protocol,* Utilisation Management Associates, Massachusetts, USA.

Victor, C., & Khahoo, A.A. (1994) Is hospital the right place? A survey of 'inappropriate' admissions to an inner London NHS Trust. *Journal of Public Health Medicine* **16**: 286–90.

Wernicke, U. (1995) Personal communication to the author by Dr Wernicke, London Health Economics Consortium.

7 ◆ Increasing the Efficiency of Clinical Service Delivery

Paul Bentley, Jonathan Asbridge, Andrew Miles,
Nicholas Price and Andreas Polychronis

Introduction

The need for improved efficacy and effectiveness has traditionally provided the most powerful motivation for changes in clinical practice. Recent changes in healthcare policies, generated largely by the needs for cost-containment, have required clinicians throughout the developed world to examine the results of their endeavours in the light of the costs incurred. Clinical effectiveness and clinical appropriateness have been examined in the preceding chapters. The efficiency of service delivery, the factors which affect it and the changes in organisational practice which may improve it, are considered here.

Efficiency and effectiveness

The distinction between effectiveness (a measure of service outcomes) and efficiency (which relates these outcomes to resource utilisation) is somewhat artificial, as an ineffective treatment or procedure cannot be efficient in terms of healthcare provision, even though it may have been delivered in an efficient manner. Similarly, an effective treatment can be rendered less effective if delivered inefficiently. We shall, however, for the purpose of this chapter, assume effectiveness and deal solely with how practice might change to achieve a greater efficiency of healthcare delivery.

The need for efficiency

Hitherto, the goal of all clinical practice, its treatments and procedures, has been to achieve the best possible outcome, whether for an individual patient or for a client group. This goal has been seen as essential and to be achieved irrespective of cost, which is not restricted to purely financial outlay; professional time and that of the patient are important factors determining efficiency. It is becoming increasingly recognised however, that the 'best possible outcome' cannot be justified at any cost. Furthermore, medical care is essentially a human activity and it is a reasonable assumption that inefficiencies will naturally exist within the process. While there is not likely to be any dissent from the concept of searching for greater efficiencies within the healthcare system, this cannot be the sole priority.

Any provider of healthcare, whether at strategic or at operational level must ensure an equitable, if not necessarily equal, service provision (Menzel 1992; Pauly 1992). However, in the application of market solutions to the problem of healthcare funding, equity of care has been seen as being potentially in conflict with the need to achieve greater efficiency (Vågerö 1994). In actual fact, promoting efficiency may lead to greater equity. The King's Fund has included efficiency (by Robert Maxwell's definition, *value for money* (Maxwell 1984)) as a quality dimension in healthcare provision. The drive for efficiency is therefore inescapable.

Is healthcare delivery any more or less efficient than other comparable activities? This may be an unfair question, but certainly between different systems worldwide there are examples of wide and extraordinary variations in spending which cannot be explained by different levels of need. In the USA, Holland and Italy, there are many more doctors per head of population than in the UK, and the expenditure on healthcare as a proportion of the gross national product shows considerable inconsistencies between countries. These differences cannot be explained by genetic or environmental factors, nor by health *per se* leading to greater or lesser needs, but more to national wealth (D'Intignano 1993). Philosophical, cultural and educational factors also modify the demand and hence dictate the supply of medical care. Nor is there necessarily any improved outcome from greater investment, indeed there is only a weak relationship between the cost and quality of care, and certainly in primary care the highest quality care may be found in a medium-cost environment (Starfield *et al.* 1994).

These differences have highlighted the potential growth in healthcare expenditure and led to the application of other mechanisms for state funding of healthcare delivery, including managed competition with a payment system designed to expand access and reduce costs (Capter 1993). With reference to these criteria it is tempting to describe the UK National Health Service as efficient. However, until the outcome of healthcare delivery achieves the same pre-eminence as the process of healthcare delivery has traditionally enjoyed, it will remain difficult to determine whether additional investment will produce returns in the form of improved efficiency.

Why increase efficiency?

In an attempt to achieve greater efficiency the NHS has been set targets through the Patient's Charter and High Level Performance Indicators. These include limits on out-patient and in-patient waiting times, the number of surgical procedure cancellations, the proportion of elective procedures performed as day cases, the proportion of new out-patient attendances and pressure to reduce the rates of non-attendance at out-patient clinics. This, undoubtedly, will improve efficiency from a patient's perspective, though whether it will lead to an overall increase in efficiency is yet to be determined. Thus, health service delivery is now subject to higher standards than have been previously achieved in the absence of additional resources being available; in other words greater efficiencies are expected.

Irrespective of these arguments, however, there is the more compelling issue of the need to maintain and to develop services, and in most countries this means within existing resources. This provides the greatest incentive for the examination of clinical practice and for the identification of areas of activity where resources can be utilised to achieve better outcomes or even released to develop new services and expand existing ones where there are unmet needs. These solutions are, theoretically, in the hands of healthcare professionals. There are, however, the additional professional and scientific reasons for the evaluation of efficiency. Limitations on junior doctors' hours, the need to provide sufficient experience and supervision to meet training requirements and the constraint on their numbers will force the need for greater efficiencies, as will be discussed. Scientific developments require the availability of additional investments in time, effort and money in order for the potential benefits to be realised. These can be met from existing resources only by the abandonment of redundant activities, yet such activities may continue unabated without the application of critical appraisal. An example would be the continued servicing of large numbers of in-patient beds originally commissioned for work now undertaken in a day-care system.

Parameters of efficiency

If improved efficiency is to be achieved through changes in practice, measures of efficiency are essential components in decision making. All procedures or treatments where the benefits outweigh the risks are deemed as necessary in the clinical setting (Capter 1993) and this leads to supply-induced demand. It is difficult to apply the usual equation of effect or output divided by energy utilisation or input to calculate efficiency in medical practice; efficiency is only a relative dimension. Costing of procedures provides a relative evaluation of unrelated services but the decision regarding the *worth* of an investigation or treatment is difficult, except when taken in the context of the available alternatives. These, however, are idealised situations and in reality it may be necessary to increase the input perhaps by a modest degree (Stehr 1993) to improve overall efficiency.

The greatest investment is in the will to change. A good example would be to increase the number of procedures undertaken during an operating theatre session by the simple expedient of appointing and deploying additional portering staff. Healthcare managers are aware of the fact that NHS traditions have not worked in this way to realise greater efficiency. The creation of additional clinical time or facility has led to increasing workload and this in turn has led to a breakdown in the process, ultimately because of greater service provision and the total costs incurred. However, if the current UK system (whereby providers are funded in proportion to work output achieved) were to work properly, this obstacle should be removed, though purchasers would find it difficult to sustain contracts under these conditions. The emphasis remains on cost containment and the achievement of the highest possible throughput, though as Miles *et al.* point out in Chapter 8, the so-called quality revolution is changing this traditional philosophy, albeit slowly, and in a manner complicated by methodological and conceptual weaknesses. Costs have therefore tended to be contained by mechanisms which lead to service limitation or rationing and the most efficient providers to not necessarily benefit directly from their efficiencies.

A strategic approach to efficiency

Given the limitations of the healthcare process there are a number of strategic issues with the potential to contribute to increased efficiency of healthcare delivery. The NHS reforms are in part clearly designed to reduce the costs of healthcare, but must avoid threats to the need for quality of care. Competition for service provision has been traditionally unacceptable to the medical profession, but now the split between health purchasers and providers, together with the creation of Trust hospitals and the increasing private sector involvement, demands greater efficiency from providers. The price for this has been an increasing bureaucracy. There is no definitive evidence which demonstrates that the extension of the market process to clinical budgeting would, or would not, make support-service users more efficient in the utilisation of resources. The introduction of high level performance indicators requires, for example, a 95% operating theatre utilisation. The Patient's Charter, for its part, determines waiting times in out-patient clinics and for urgent and non-urgent in-patient surgery, representing a further example of government pressure in response to political needs to effect efficiency savings.

The NHS reforms have undoubtedly created a new climate in acute hospitals, largely as a result of change in philosophy in the management of acute hospitals. They have also removed obstacles to hospital access, such as the referral system, out-patient in-patient waiting times, transport arrangements and even car parking provision, to encourage the referral and treatment of larger numbers of patients. In the UK, purchasers are examining healthcare needs and will undoubtedly identify essential areas of provision. More particularly, they will identify those procedures which have been developed but which are non-essential and might therefore no longer be provided at all within the NHS. Some procedures should be deliberately excluded from NHS funding (such as those undertaken for minor cosmetic purposes), without any reduction in the health of the population. This will liberate resources needed to preserve essential activities. The mechanisms by which these decisions can be made have proven elusive, although purchasers are now turning to scientifically derived evidence of effectiveness to help with their strategies.

Translating these initiatives into practice is difficult (Scott & Jackson 1995). The major obstacle has been in putting changes into practice, even when the evidence for potentially improved outcomes and greater efficiency is available. In this context the value of health promotion and screening programmes will require extremely careful evaluation to determine whether investment in them will prove to be an efficient use of resources. Mass chest radiography for tuberculosis detection became archaic when the low detection rate was identified in the 1950s. Screening for cervical cancer and more recently breast cancer will need to be subject to the same evaluation formerly undertaken after the necessary level of experience has been acquired, but already doubts about the efficiency of these programmes are being expressed (Kikuchi & Inaba 1992; Raffle *et al.* 1995), although disappointing outcomes may be more a function of inappropriate objectives (Skegg 1995). This is despite the enormous public pressures for funded screening programmes to be extended.

Comprehensive health screens, that is those programmes not specifically aimed at a single disease or condition, are of even more dubious value in terms of disease prevention. These may, however, provide a very worthwhile function in excluding a range of disorders or disabilities by providing qualified reassurance to the patient. The cost of more targeted programmes, such as mammography, may still be very high and inefficient unless optimal results are achieved (Breen & Brown 1994) but when programmes have several component tests, there are also scientific and logistical problems (Faivre *et al.* 1991; Kikuchi & Inaba 1992). Health promotion programmes provided by employers have shown considerable cost benefits when measured over several years (Golaszewski *et al.* 1992). This is seen as an effective return on investment, a mechanism perhaps not yet available to healthcare providers. Only pre-natal care for poor women, tests in newborns for some congenital disorders and childhood immunisation have been shown to be cost effective. Screening for cancer and hypertension may cost more than the treatment for these conditions once they come to medical attention (Leutwyler 1995). Massive investment in screening programmes therefore threatens the global efficiency of healthcare by diversion of resources.

Integration of primary and secondary healthcare delivery

The primary–secondary care interface has been considered in Chapters 1, 3 and 4, in terms of the utility of the audit mechanism in securing a so-called 'seamless service'. Suffice it here to note that initiatives for closer integration of primary and secondary healthcare systems offer a great opportunity for more healthcare provision by increasing the speed and appropriateness of referral and discharge. Since the 1960s direct access for the patient to coronary care units for diagnosis and management of chest pain, oncology units for neutropenic fever and haemophilia units for acute bleeding, whether by self-referral or via the emergency ambulance service, has created trends toward patient-focused or at least disease-centred care. More recently, open access for patients with haematuria, rectal bleeding or chest pain has allowed patients with potentially significant symptoms requiring urgent investigation and treatment to be seen by a specialist, thereby circumventing many traditional routes of referral with consequent savings in time and money. The price of this, as always claimed by supporters of the primary care 'gatekeeper' function, will be an inappropriate referral rate and the dangers of the specialist being obliged to deal with problems for which he is not trained. It is possible that the gatekeeping function may shift to become located more closely to secondary care providers. The clinical audit mechanism remains central to the identification and correction of the inefficiencies of the primary–secondary care interface (Miles *et al.* 1996). See also Miles *et al.* in Chapters 1, 2 and 3 of this volume.

Centralisation of healthcare delivery

The centralisation of services has been used as a means to increase efficiency after many years of change during which services have been increasingly decentralised closer to the patient's locality. Centralisation is particularly valuable where clinical services are highly dependent on other specialised support services (e.g. intensive care, radiology, pathology). It has now resulted in a transfer of the burden of transport and accommodation to the patient. There must, however, be an optimal size or volume of work for any services to remain viable and competent and there has been a growing realisation that increasing volumes ultimately do not lead to an economy of scale. However, high cost and labour-intensive services such as cardiac surgery, vascular surgery, neurosurgery, medical oncology and in-patient psychiatry need to be centralised for reasons other than practical economy. The shortage of specialist trained staff, the need to maintain a level of expertise through practice and the provision of training and education facilities will require that medical skills are concentrated rather than dispersed.

If the value of centralised single-specialty services is to be properly realised, it is essential that there be a change in the working philosophy of the consultants involved. Traditionally, a consultant has been an independent practitioner providing care of a standard defined largely by himself and making decisions based on his own education and personal experience. These can be highly inefficient in the absence of established standards and protocols of care to overcome the wide variation in practices (Burns *et al.* 1994; Scott & Jackson 1995). Where more than one consultant is providing a specialist service, it is going to be difficult, though absolutely essential, that there be a high level of standardisation and management of patients through the application of agreed protocols of care. These are seen as a major threat by many specialists, but properly constructed protocols should allow considerable opportunity for a consultant still to use his skills and judgement and spend less of his time on tasks beneath his skill level. The concept of clinical judgement can only be seen as valuable when the patient's best interest is served rather than the doctor's whim. Indeed, as Rigge points out in Chapter 11 of this volume, many consultants have 'an excessive regard for the sanctity of clinical freedom'. The concept of case management and development of critical pathways for patient groups will be discussed in this context later in this chapter.

Operational efficiency

Referrals from primary care

The current system of hospital referral particularly to named consultants impairs patient access to specialist services, creates the possibility of uneven workloads for consultants and generates waiting lists. A more accessible and therefore more efficient process would be referral by telephone to a consultant who then has the power to decide whether prior investigations need to be undertaken or urgent referral arranged. Kassirer (1994) considers that primary care physicians may in this way reduce the number of specialist visits by broadening the scope of the care they provide and consulting with specialists themselves more readily. It would then be necessary for a consultant service to be available for consultation with patients every week day.

This approach, which need not necessarily be led initially by a consultant medical practitioner, could be built using the case management concept described by Davenport and Noreer (1994). They reviewed a number of American corporations where case management provided a way to increase organisation efficiency, timeliness and customer satisfaction. Shapiro *et al.* (1992) identified case management as particularly useful in processes that deal with customers which involve managing an entire cycle of activity, from customer order to product or service delivery, billing and payment. In clinical terms this would be a team leader who deals with referrals which involve rapid assessment, investigation, treatment and referral back to primary healthcare teams. In the market-led NHS this would involve ensuring the contract department receive the information in order to send bills either to purchasing health authorities or to GP fundholders.

Inter-functional co-ordination of healthcare professionals and high consumer service levels

Harrington (1991) discusses the concept of business process improvement. Process thinking implies a structure based on outcomes rather than on functional skills or reporting relationships. The existing hierarchy in medical practice, both in hospitals and on the GP–consultant interfaces causes barriers to be put in place which detract from the efficiency required by an increasingly cash-limited health service. This is coupled with the paternalistic grace and favour structures of most NHS institutions which is based on the traditional division of labour and its inherent lack of customer responsiveness. Most hospitals are administered for the convenience of the staff who work in them rather than for the patients who are referred to them.

Davenport (1995) refers to this lack of responsiveness in areas where assembly line models of production are in place which are not well suited to problem-solving interfunctional co-ordination and high customer service levels. He cites the development of cross functional teams for certain types of tasks and a system which meets his case management needs in a structure based on relatively independent functional experts, such as scientists in a research-orientated organisation or physicians in the hospital. Davenport refers to these as functional experts but does not believe they are efficient at permanent task execution, particularly of highly structured tasks. The cardiologist, for example, is excellent in the diagnosis and management of heart failure but is not necessarily adept at ensuring that the patient's orthopaedic and psychological problems are addressed. Functional specialists are also often better at 'practising their specialty than at providing service to customers' as the patients of many physicians will attest. Davenport (1995) identifies five alternatives to work organisation and tasks requirement but views that the benefit of case management is its flexibility in the handling of multiple tasks.

The development of critical pathways and clinical protocols for most patient groups would enable the general practitioner (GP) to access a non-medical case manager. Rapid ordering of investigations could then take place with a decision by the GP as to whether, on the information gained from the results of investigations, referral to a consultant medical practitioner is necessary, or whether the results of investigations allow the GP to continue treating the patients against clinical protocols developed by experts in the field. This might be particularly useful in the treatment of emergency admissions to hospitals where many patients are sent for rapid assessment and investigation and require admission, not so much for medical care, but for nursing care which could be provided in neighbourhood hospitals or with support in the patient's own home.

Waiting lists and waiting times

Under current arrangements waiting lists have tended to create a rationing of healthcare, with a proportion of patients ultimately not attending for treatment. This may contribute to the 'did not attend' rate which has reached substantial proportions in some clinics, with consequent waste of out-patient consultation time, in-patient accommodation and operating theatre time in particular. There is no operational need for waiting lists with any significant associated patient waiting time; if a waiting list is stable then patients are being added at the same rate as they are being removed (either by receiving treatment or no longer requiring such advice or treatment which may be offered). Such waiting lists should be capable of elimination by a single initiative and thereafter not recur.

Rising waiting lists are an indication for greater investment in clinical time. Thus careful monitoring of waiting lists, or more properly waiting times, should be used to manage and eliminate waiting lists wherever they exist. However, out-patient referrals may be arranged for a variety of reasons. A proportion of patients will have known conditions requiring specialist advice or treatment beyond the scope of the GP's normal practice, and may be managed as above. Others will not have an established diagnosis but are known to have a medical problem. There will, however, be a substantial number of patients referred without there being any expected outcome other than the reassurance that no significant disorder is causing their symptoms. These patients may have their anxieties relieved by a second opinion but will be seen, in terms of medical activity, as valueless. This may appear inefficient, though from a patient's perspective the outcome will be extremely valued, as emphasised in Chapter 11.

Out-patients management

The need for follow-up out-patient attendances and the interval between them have never been defined. Several studies have demonstrated considerable yet unexplained variation in the intervals between scheduled consultations (Lichtenstein *et al.* 1986; Petitti & Grumbach 1993). Primary care physicians tend to see patients more frequently than their colleagues in hospital-based practice. This may reflect differences in experience and suggests that hospital clinics are more efficient, though these clinics are more expensive to run than an average GP surgery. Remarkable improvements in efficiency can be achieved by adjustment of appointment times in relation to the patient's real needs (Jennings 1991).

It is frequently difficult to identify, particularly in the treatment and monitoring of chronic disorders, how often a patient needs to be seen in an out-patient clinic. The major factors which determine this are the often misplaced concern of a doctor wishing not to appear to have overlooked the cause, an unresolved problem, or even insufficient confidence on the part of the doctor to change from the interval since the previous consultation. Purchasers, however, may apply pressure by funding only a limited number of re-attendances, though such interventions are unevaluated and potentially dangerous (Miles *et al.* 1995).

Any patients with defined problems such as ischaemic heart disease, diabetes, hypertension, bleeding or thrombotic disorders, cancer and leukaemia are managed in specialist clinics to which they may have direct access. The efficiency of many of these clinics is yet to be measured, but is likely to exceed that of more general clinics by streamlining a new process to provide a more patient-focused service. These facilities run the risk of assuming all responsibility for the patient's care irrespective of the relevance of any additional clinical problem creating difficulties for the specialist who may feel obliged to provide care for disorders outside her normal practice.

Outreach clinics

The advent of fundholding general practices has created a demand for clinics previously conducted in hospital out-patient departments to be transferred to the GP's own premises. This may be soundly economical for the cost-conscious GP and for the patient who receives advice and treatment locally, but cannot be considered efficient in terms of the use of a consultant's time (London 1995). Fewer patients will be seen, with consequent periods of service inactivity and reduction in expertise. Scheduling will be complicated if clinics are to be attended by only referred patients; emergency referrals will be difficult to accommodate, travelling time for consultants will increase, access to support facilities (for example, pathology, radiology and physiotherapy) will be impaired, and the need for some hospital referrals will remain. Consultants will be taken from their hospital base, and hospital clinics – which are staffed with junior doctors who attend for training – will be undermined. If those junior doctors were instead to attend the general practitioner's clinic alongside the consultant, their training would be limited.

The admission process

The escalating numbers of emergency admissions will increase the risk of unnecessary or inappropriate admissions. In terms of medical manpower greater utilisation may lead to apparent increases in efficiency as the number of medical staff employed generally is not related to workload. However, staff overloaded with inappropriate duties will become *ipso facto* inefficient. All emergency admission units must equip themselves to provide a second opinion facility supported with simple diagnostic tests, without necessarily being obliged to admit the patient. Early pregnancy assessment units and chest pain clinics are excellent examples of how skilled staff and technical facilities can be deployed to the efficient provision of advice and, where necessary, further referral or management of specific conditions, thus creating high-volume workloads where a substantial proportion of patients do not require admission to hospital.

In-patient management

The creation of admissions wards would concentrate medical activities where urgently admitted patients are in greatest need. This would also improve quality by avoiding disruption of other wards. Junior doctors should be educated in the use of correspondence and other media as effective means of communication.

Critical pathways

The use of critical pathways in the achievement of clinical goals in a timely and efficient manner has been examined in a number of centres in the USA, Australia and the UK (Johnson 1994; Kitchiner *et al*. 1996). The increase in efficiency identified by these authors includes, for example, a reduction in length of stay from 16 days to 10 days for total hip replacements (Johnson 1994).

Improvements in efficiency can be created by the design of set patterns of care for defined procedures. Increases in efficiency have been identified in such areas as door-to-needle times for fibrinolytic therapy in patients suffering myocardial infarction (Johnson 1994), reduction in the duration of intravenous antibiotic therapy from a consensus opinion on the optimum length of time for which they should be given (Johnson 1994) and the reduction of assisted ventilation time following cardiac surgery (Hoffman 1993).

Other improvements created by the use of critical pathways were reductions in the complication rate following coronary artery by-pass grafting, from 16.6% to 5% (Hoffman 1993), and an improvement in the satisfaction of patients with the information they received by continually refining the education and interventions on the path in the light of regular surveying of the patient's views. The most valuable component of the development of critical pathways for patients, based on objective evidence, clinical guidelines and business process re-engineering, is the development of the multidisciplinary clinical team which has responsibility for ensuring the management of the patient's care from before admission to after discharge. The first step in developing critical pathways is to develop a consensus between all practitioners for the most appropriate way that a patient should be managed.

There is no place for tribalism in the efficiency-focused NHS. Simpson (1994) states that doctors are not traditionally strong corporate team players; the nature of their profession with ultimate named responsibility for individual patients dictates an organisation of single players, albeit supported by their own teams of juniors. This means that many doctors gain little experience of working as equal players in teams. It is clear that there is a particular need to examine team working and communication across disciplines and this needs to be incorporated into the training of medical students. The doctor's team work is essentially part of the preparation for all other members of the interdisciplinary professions who work with patients in acute hospitals and primary care. It is ironic that the one professional group which sees itself as being the natural leader of these teams finds it very difficult to work in a team or to accept that other members of the team have a useful contribution to make. The reader is referred to Kitchiner *et al*.

(1996) for a useful review of the basic principles and practice associated with critical pathways.

Clinical algorithms

Clinical algorithms, whereby options for the management of a patient are presented in response to certain findings or observations, have many applications and could increase the efficiency of service delivery (Neale & Chang 1991; Ament & Hasman 1993) by establishing a uniform approach to diagnosis and treatment without undermining the need for decisions essential to the patient's management. This is distinct from the fully developed critical care pathways which require a more rigid adherence to an agreed protocol for specific components of the patient's care. If properly applied they are demonstrably effective and both doctors and nurses find them helpful (Grimshaw *et al.* 1995). They have, however, been applied in only a limited fashion, perhaps because of unjustified fears on the part of consultants that they may interfere with clinical decision making. Indeed, the algorithm, however skilfully constructed, must allow for the immense variability in clinical expression of disease and its response to treatment. This emphasises, rather than obviates, the centrality of clinical judgement (Feinstein 1994).

Ward rounds

Ward rounds are a traditional way of providing in-patient care. The substantial resource utilisation, certainly in terms of the medical time consumed, indicates that ward rounds are grossly inefficient. Without them, however, there would be no focus for medical decision making and substantial training opportunities would be lost (although there may be appropriate ways of substituting for these). Farag and Tinker (1985) have shown that ward rounds have the capacity to delay discharge in a significant number of patients, and they recommended instead daily visits by consultants to the wards. Some authors regard the traditional ward round as more symbolic than effective (Bulstrode 1995) and no longer capable of providing the continuity of care for which it was originally intended.

Medical staffing

In the UK there have been new and considerable pressures on medical staffing levels for several years originating, perhaps, in the inadequate career prospects of newly qualified doctors. This difficulty is compounded by a recent requirement for the British system to come into line with EC training schemes and the need to achieve mutual recognition of individual state qualifications. Evaluation of the UK system culminated in the Calman (1993) report. This focuses on training without consideration of service provision and the continual reductions in junior doctors' hours will reduce further the manpower available to the health service.

The impact of these measures could be considerable (Jones *et al.* 1992), and the medical 'firm' may become the first victim of the need to use the services of junior doctors more efficiently with continuity of care provided by some new structure (Bulstrode 1995); indeed the need for patient care to pass from one doctor to another may conceivably improve case review and consequently the quality of care (Bulstrode 1995). There have been no restrictions in consultants' hours and as they are no longer formally training, there could be a considerable transfer of work, both routine and emergency, to consultant medical staff. Consultants' contracts and job plans could be modified to achieve this. However, one of the obligations of consultants is to supervise junior doctors in training. Furthermore, there is a considerable recruitment problem, particularly in some specialties; in anaesthetics for example, where many consultant posts remain vacant throughout the UK.

The need to meet training requirements endangers the efficient delivery of care in the short term. A service provided only by consultants could, with adequate and appropriate support, become considerably more efficient than the present service provided through the hierarchical system which characterises most medical 'firms'. Certainly, the contribution of the pre-registration house officer is being questioned and future constraints on medical manpower, with consequent restructuring, may negate the need for these posts. This will impact on the level of skill of medical graduates, who may be expected to have a higher level of capability and acumen at the start of their careers. The deployment of nurse practitioners (Snyder *et al.* 1994), especially in highly specialised areas of work, can improve efficiency. The appropriateness of tasks undertaken by doctors and nurses therefore requires continuous critical review.

Medical records

Clinicians are necessarily obsessive about record keeping, though they seldom agree on content and format. As storage of bulky paper-based systems becomes increasingly difficult and the complexity of modern healthcare requires the provision of simultaneous access to a number of users, the need to find an alternative storage medium becomes imperative. The problems encountered with the use of paper-based systems include the factors listed below:

- transport costs
- losses of items from casenotes
- poor legibility
- important information is difficult to identify quickly
- the absence of vital information is difficult to detect
- information is accessible to only a single user at a time, yet the

health record is the sole repository of information central to the management of both the patient and the healthcare facility

- the work of different health professionals is often duplicated, which leads to increased costs, perpetuation of errors and duplication of information.

The recent report of the Audit Commission (1995) indicates that existing medical records systems are generally inadequate to meet the requirements of the modern health service. One way by which this problem could be overcome would be the development of an integrated medical record to which all health professionals would contribute. This has worked well in maternity and ITU departments, and has been introduced in general surgery in conjunction with critical pathways of care in some general hospitals.

The development of the electronic medical record is a natural progression from the increased use of automation in information collection and processing in the health service. Starting from the principle that the medical record should guide treatment and should facilitate effective management of clinical risk, an electronic, self-checking record system will eliminate duplication and avoid the perpetuation of errors. It could assist clinicians in the management of complexity, for example by automatically issuing warnings of drug interactions and by highlighting when the planned care has not been delivered. Such an innovation would lead to increased efficiency and safer clinical practice. Further advantages would include reduced storage and retrieval costs and improved access to patient information. Software development is therefore indicated to ensure that an electronic medical record could be maintained virus-free, tamper-proof, protected against loss and be legible, while maintaining confidentiality. It would also be possible to trace medication, individual prostheses and implants, facilitate audit and enable the recall of patients to become swifter and more accurate. Greater accuracy in costing healthcare would be achieved.

The launch of the new NHS number together with increased access for healthcare providers to the NHS Administrative Register means that patients could soon be identifiable in any healthcare location, and information of greatly improved quality will be available for clinical activity and epidemiological study. The first obstacle to overcome in the achievement of the fully electronic medical record is the lack of short-term finance, as the enormous cost savings will only be realised in the long term.

The mechanism by which health providers fund major investments in technology in order to achieve the level of information required by them to operate more efficiently needs urgent consideration. Current approaches lead to an over-cumbersome system with low productivity and consequent demoralisation. In addition, considerable cultural change will be necessary, not only for the introduction of information technology (IT) systems but also to create the acceptability of healthcare professionals other than doctors contributing productively to a single record. This, after all, shakes the foundations of the cultural paradigm that doctors are the only professional group fitted to provide primary levels of care. The impact of an electronic medical record upon skill mix cannot be overestimated as it will reduce the requirement for clerical and administrative staff, as well as affecting the balance of skilled medical and nursing staff to greater numbers of semi-skilled staff on hospital wards.

Management of change

Introducing change of this type requires careful management if it is successfully to avoid resistance. Considerable amounts of the management literature have been devoted to the planning and management of change. A key element to consider during the development of a new medical records system is user involvement during the design and implementation stages rather than leaving these tasks in the hands of IT specialists. Communication with the staff during all stages of project development is essential as the effects of change will be widespread and could have a major impact on their working lives. Piloting and modelling are essentially to improve any system's credibility and remove any flaws. Once established, however, electronic systems rapidly prove their worth by their fidelity and speed of access to information. A simple example would be the improvements in blood banking by a computer's search capability, by which previous records could be checked and incorrect samples identified. This is impossible with a paper-based record.

Certainly, in terms of hospital management, the transport of large numbers of files from one location to another, the mechanism of filing, retrieval and long-term storage of paper-based records, would all be overcome. Furthermore, patients could be equipped with a reduced format copy of the record themselves and could produce this, should they be seeking medical advice in another location. In addition to direct patient management, an electronic medical record system would produce enormous benefits in terms of epidemiological study, needs assessment and costing of individual patient care. The obstacles to introducing these systems are largely financial, as they require a substantial investment followed by an enormous cultural change within the organisation. The problems of compliance tend to resolve with time and the quality of medical record keeping improves (Holnloser & Soltanian 1994). Clearly, the existing medical records departments would view such a development as a serious threat and clinical staff may well perceive using an IT facility as an alteration of their role. However, it is common experience within clinical areas, for example radiology departments and pathology laboratories, that computer-based records are becoming an essential part of the workings of the system.

Information technology

There are now many areas of clinical activity where management could be more efficient with the application of computerised systems. They include the following:

- operating theatre scheduling (Bottini *et al.* 1994)
- diagnosis (Velanovich 1994)
- medical imaging (Orphanoudakis *et al.* 1994)
- decision making (Heathfield *et al.* 1991; Nelson & Gardner 1993; Aliferis *et al.* 1994)
- vital signs records (Raygor 1994)
- information (Regan 1991)
- word processing (Ecker 1991)
- medical records (Stetson *et al.* 1991; Jackson *et al.* 1994)
- quality assurance (Aghababian *et al.* 1992)
- staff deployment (Hu 1993)
- anticoagulant dosing (Hunt 1993)
- bar coding for drug usage evaluation (Zarowitz *et al.* 1993)
- deployment of nurse practitioners (Snyder *et al.* 1994) and para-medical obstetric staff (Hibbard *et al.* 1993).

Conclusion

The environment in which healthcare is being delivered is dynamic and developing, where today's decisions have to be made with one eye on the map of tomorrow. Creating systems which can meet today's needs and those of tomorrow requires careful strategic thought if the investment of time and money is to be safeguarded. It is likely that the need for greater efficiency will remain a feature of clinical practice. This should be seen as a stimulus for re-evaluating all aspects of care provision. It has been difficult to identify an area of clinical practice where efficiency could not be improved and the authors would like to feel that the instances identified here are only examples offered to initiate a process which should become incorporated into every practitioner's approach to his work.

References

Aghababian, R.V., Williams, K.A., Holbrook, J.A. & Lew, R. (1992) Computer applications in quality assurance. *Emergency Medicine Clinics of North America* **10**: 627–47.

Aliferis, C.F., Cooper, G.F. & Bankowitz, R. (1994) A temporal analysis of QMR: abstracted temporal representation and reasoning and initial assessment of diagnostic performance trade-offs. *Proceedings – the Annual Symposium on Computer Applications in Medical Care*, Washington, DC, pp. 709–15.

Ament, A. & Hasman, A. (1993) Optimal test strategy in the case of two tests and one disease. *International Journal of Bio-Medical Computing* **33**: 179–97.

Audit Commission (1995) *Setting the Records Straight – A Study of Hospital Medical Records*, HMSO, London.

Bottini, A.G., Priest, J.G., Murray, R., Wiley, P.D., Moore, K., Smith, B. & Crandall, D.B. (1994) Development of a user-defined surgical database using a personal computer network. *Military Medicine* **159**: 571–6.

Breen, N. & Brown, M.L. (1994) The price of mammography in the United States: data from the National Survey of Mammography Facilities. *Milbank Quarterly* **72**: 431–50.

Bulstrode, C. (1995) Continuity of care – sacred cow or vital necessity? *British Medical Journal* **310**: 1144–5.

Burns, L.R., Chilingerian, J.A. & Wholey, D.R. (1994) The effect of physician practice organization on efficient utilization of hospital resources. *Health Services Research* **29**: 583–603.

Calman, K. (1993) *The Calman Report*, HMSO, London.

Capter, P. (1993) Managed competition that works. *Journal of the American Medical Association* **269**: 2524–6.

Davenport, C. (1995) Responsiveness and co-ordination in clinical care. *British Medical Journal* **310**: 996–9.

Davenport, C. & Noreer, A. (1994) Critical pathways – the pivotal tool. *Journal of Cardiovascular Nursing* **7**: 30–37.

D'Intignano, M. (1993) Financing of health care in Europe. In *Health Care Reforms in Europe. Proceedings of the First Meeting of the Working Party of Health Care Reforms in Europe* (ed. C. Artundo, C. Sabellarides and H. Vuori), World Health Organization Regional Office for Europe, Copenhagen.

Ecker, R.I. (1991) Word processing in the physician's office. *Seminars in Dermatology* **10**: 107–11.

Faivre, J., Arveux, P., Milan, C., Durand, G., Lamour, J. & Bedenne, L. (1991) Participation in mass screening for colorectal cancer: results of screening and rescreening from the Burgundy study. *European Journal of Cancer Prevention* **1**: 49–55.

Farag, R.R. & Tinker, G.M. (1985) Delay in discharge of patients from an acute geriatric unit. *Health Trends* **17**: 41.

Feinstein, A. (1994) Clinical judgement re-visited: the distraction of quantitative models. *Annals of Internal Medicine* **120**: 799–805.

Golaszewski, T., Snow, D., Lynch, W., Yen, L. & Solomita, D. (1992) A benefit-to-cost analysis of a work-site health promotion program. *Journal of Occupational Medicine* **34**: 1164–72.

Grimshaw, J., Eccles, M. & Russell, I. (1995) Developing clinically valid practice guidelines. *Journal of Evaluation in Clinical Practice* **1**: 37–48.

Harrington, A. (1991) An introduction to critical paths. *Quality Management in Health Care* **1**: 45–54.

Heathfield, H.A., Winstanley, G. & Kirkham, N. (1991) Decision support system for the differential diagnosis of breast disease. *Journal of Biomedical Engineering* **13**: 51–7.

Hibbard, B.M., Dawson, A., Boyce, J., Oliver, M., Goodall, K., Organ, P. & Rookes, N. (1993) A paramedic based emergency domiciliary obstetric service: the South Glamorgan experience. *British Journal of Obstetrics and Gynaecology* **100**: 618–22.

Holnloser, A. & Soltanian, N. (1994) Obtaining information from medical records. *Journal of the Royal College of Physicians* **8**: 267–75.

Hu, S.C. (1993) Computerized monitoring of emergency department patient flow. *American Journal of Emergency Medicine* **11**: 8–11.

Hunt, B. (1993) Development of a MUMPS-based anticoagulant management system. *British Journal of Biomedical Science* **50**: 117–24.

Jackson, K.I., Gibby, G.L., van der Aa, J.J., Arroyo, A.A. & Gravenstein, J.S. (1994) The efficiency of preoperative evaluation: a comparison of computerized and paper recording systems. *Journal of Clinical Monitoring* **10**: 189–93.

Jennings, M. (1991) Audit of a new appointments system in a hospital outpatient clinic. *British Medical Journal* **302**: 148–9.

Johnson, S. (1994) Pathway to the heart of care quality. *Nursing Management* **1**: 26–7.

Jones, J., Sanderson, C. & Black, N. (1992) What will happen to the quality of care with fewer junior doctors? A Delphi study of consultant physicians' views. *Journal of the Royal College of Physicians of London* **26**: 36–40.

Kassirer, J. (1994) Access to specialty care. *New England Journal of Medicine* **331**: 1151–3.

Kikuchi, S. & Inaba, T. (1992) Problems associated with mass-screening system for gastric cancer in Japan. *Japanese Journal of Public Health* **39**: 380–86.

Kitchiner, D., Davidson, C. & Bundred, P. (1996) Integrated care pathways: effective tools for continuous evaluation of clinical practice. *Journal of Evaluation in Clinical Practice* **2**: 65–9.

Leutwyler, K. (1995) The price of prevention. *Scientific American* **259**: 99–103.

Lichtenstein, M.J., Sweetnman, P.M. & Elwood, P.C. (1986) Visit frequency for controlled essential hypertension: several practitioners' opinions. *Journal of Family Practice* **23**: 331–6.

London, D. (1995) Reaching out is hard to do. *Health Service Journal* **15**: 89.

Maxwell, R.J. (1984) Quality assessment in health. *British Medical Journal* **288**: 1470–72.

Menzel, P.T. (1992) Equality, autonomy, and efficiency: what health care system should we have? *Journal of Medicine and Philosophy* **17**: 32–57.

Miles, A., Bentley, D.P., Grey, J. & Polychronis, A. (1995) Purchasing quality in clinical practice: what on earth do we mean? *Journal of Evaluation in Clinical Practice* **1**: 87–95.

Miles, A., Bentley, D.P., Price, N., Polychronis, A., Grey, J. & Asbride, J. (1996) The total healthcare audit system: a systematic methodology for clinical practice evaluation and development in NHS provider organisations. *Journal of Evaluation in Clinical Practice* **2**: 37–64.

Neale, E.J. & Chang, A.M. (1991) Clinical algorithms. *Medical Teacher* **13**: 317–22.

Nelson, B.D. & Gardner, R.M. (1993) Decision support for concurrent utilization review using a HELP-embedded expert system. *Proceedings – The Annual Symposium on Computer Applications in Medical Care*, Washington, DC, pp. 176–82.

Orphanoudakis, S.C., Chronaki, C. & Kostomanolakis, S. (1994) 12C: a system for the indexing, storage and retrieval of medical images by content. *Medical Informatics* **19**: 109–22.

Pauly, M.V. (1992) Fairness and feasibility in national health care systems. *Health Economics* **1**: 93–103.

Petitti, D.B. & Grumbach, K. (1993) Variation in physicians' recommendations about revisit interval for three common conditions. *Journal of Family Practice* **37**: 235–40.

Raffle, A.E., Alden, B. & Mackenzie, E.F.D. (1995) Detection rates for abnormal cervical smears: what are we screening for? *Lancet* **345**: 1469–73.

Raygor, A.J. (1994) A study of the paper chart and its potential for computerization. *Computers in Nursing* **12**: 23–8.

Regan, B.G. (1991) Computerised information exchange in health care. *Medical Journal of Australia* **154**: 140–44.

Scott, T. & Jackson, P. (1995) Using information for managing clinical services effectively. *British Medical Journal* **310**, 848–50.

Shapiro, M., Richards, J.S. & Baldwin, P.J. (1992) Critical pathway methodology. *Annals of Thoracic Surgery* **58**: 57–65.

Simpson, N. (1994) Specialists in the United States, what lessons? *British Medical Journal* **310**: 724–7.

Skegg, D.C.G. (1995) Cervical screening blues. *Lancet* **345**: 1451–2.

Snyder, J.V., Sirio, C.A., Angus, D.C., Hravnak, M.T., Kobert, S.N., Sinz, E.H. & Rudy, E.B. (1994) Trial of nurse practitioners in intensive care. *New Horizons* **2**: 296–304.

Starfield, B., Powe, N.R., Weiner, J.R., Stuart, M., Steinwachs, D., Scholle, S.H. & Gerstenberger, A. (1994) Costs vs quality in different types of primary care settings. *Journal of the American Medical Association* **272**: 1903–1908.

Stehr, H. (1993) Economic and structural aspects of modern medical technology. *Aktuelle Radiologie* **3**: 323–9.

Stetson, D.M., Eberhart, R.C., Dobbins, R.W. & Pugh, W. (1991) Medical Practice Support System. A medical practitioner's multimedia workstation. *Proceedings – The Annual Symposium on Computer Applications in Medical Care*, Washington, DC, pp. 932–4.

Vågerö, D. (1994) Equity and efficiency in health reform. A European view. *Social Science and Medicine* **39**: 1203–10.

Velanovich, V. (1994) Bayesian analysis in the diagnostic process. *American Journal of Medical Quality* **9**: 158–61.

Zarowitz, B., Petitta, A., Mlynarek, M., Touchette, M., Peters, M., Long, P. & Patel, R. (1993) Bar-code technology applied to drug-use evaluation. *American Journal of Hospital Pharmacy* **50**: 935–9.

8 ◆ Purchasing Quality in Clinical Practice: Precedents and Problems

Andrew Miles, Paul Bentley, Nicholas Price and Andreas Polychronis

Introduction

Traditional healthcare philosophy has promoted the contention that 'the more health care provided, the better' (Sheldon & Borowitz 1993). Patient throughput has therefore represented the pre-eminent concern of NHS management, with the 'quality' of care representing a secondarily considered component of healthcare delivery. The so-called 'quality revolution', despite its employment of imperfect definitions and the use of methodologies of widely differing rationale and effectiveness (Miles 1995a, b; Loughlin 1993; 1994; 1995), has precipitated a major change in this thinking. The central philosophy of the UK government is now explicit in requiring the care delivered within the NHS to be of 'good quality', as Miles *et al.* discuss in Chapter 1 of this volume.

A fundamental difficulty, notwithstanding that of definition, has been of a strategic nature; the identification and selection of methodologies which can characterise existing practice, introduce recommended changes and demonstrate quantifiable increases in such central dimensions of the quality of clinical care as effectiveness, appropriateness and efficiency. The NHS reforms have aimed at achieving such a position through the creation of an internal market in which the responsibility for purchasing services has been separated from the responsibility for providing them (Robinson 1994). While some authors heralded this event as the birth of a new, efficient, effective and appropriate service, others disagreed. Consider Charlton (1993):

'... the reforms have enhanced control from both the bureaucratic and market mechanisms at the expense of professional influence.* The result has been a complex, contradictory and probably unstable mixture of purchaser–provider splits in which self-governing NHS trust hospitals work alongside units directly managed by the purchasers, while traditional primary healthcare teams live next door to fundholding practices with both purchaser and provider functions. And into this state of evolving chaos, the NHS hierarchy is attempting to inject long-term planning, strategic thinking, and priorities, through *The Health of the Nation'*.

*see also Bunker (1994)

Central to the strategic development of the purchasing function was the advice promulgated in *Working for Patients* (Secretaries of State for Health UK 1989) which described two models for healthcare commissioning. The first focused on the role of the district health authority and the second on the role of GPs. The White Paper envisaged that health authorities would employ epidemiological and related techniques in the assessment of health needs and, on the basis of its results, purchase a corresponding range of healthcare services for the local population for which it was responsible. Such commissioning would exclude those healthcare services controlled by GP fundholders who were extended the authority to purchase a rather more limited range of services in direct response to the demands of their patients. There is therefore, as Ham (1994) points out, a quintessential difference between these two purchasing functions, with needs-based purchasing exercised by health authorities and demand-based purchasing exercised by GP fundholders. In reality, these two entities have employed differing approaches to the purchasing function which 'seek to combine the leverage of health authorities with the bite of fundholders' (Ham 1994; Shapiro 1994).

Ham (1994) describes this interaction as involving those functions listed below:

- general practitioners giving advice to District Health Authorities
- locality purchasing
- practice sensitive purchasing
- fundholding consortia
- general practitioner multi-funds
- total general practitioner fundholding.

Ham observes the spontaneous emergence of these functions as resulting from the synthesis of policy in a 'bottom up', rather than 'top down' approach. This author views such diversity as essentially positive in that, through stimulation of change, it has precipitated a culture of competition between purchasing authorities, with each attempting to demonstrate its superiority in the overall improvement of clinical services in provider organisations. There has been, however, a risk of fragmentation where approaches employed by health authorities have been insufficiently co-ordinated with those being taken by GP fundholders.

Such poor co-ordination, where it has occurred and though undesirable, was of limited significance given that the fundholding function was initially limited to a relatively small number of GP practices. The expansion of the fundholding function has risked the danger of duplication as the advent of an integrated approach to purchasing between health authorities and GPs occurred in parallel with the development of the GP fundholding function (Ham 1994). The further development of the NHS purchasing function (Beecham 1994; NHSME 1994a) has placed great emphasis on purchasing led within the primary healthcare setting and it appears likely that the number of fundholding practices in existence in 1994/5 will double by 1997/8, establishing the fundholder purchasing function as a permanent feature of the NHS.

The role of the purchasing mechanism in the development of quality in provider clinical practice is in need of urgent research and clarification. Indeed, it is acknowledged that the commissioning function is in need of considerable development (Gill 1993; Kirkup & Donaldson 1994; Rumsey *et al.* 1994) and this is proving difficult for the former health authorities given the substantial increase in the prominence of the GP fundholding initiative (NHSME 1994a). Colleagues are aware of the executive power managers have gained within the newly reformed NHS. What are the reasons which contraindicate the exercise of this authority to regulate formerly unregulated clinicians and to preclude 'sluggish or uneducated clinicians' persisting in 'old fashioned and eccentric practices under the guise of clinical freedom' (Charlton 1993)? The approach to dealing with such clinicians at the time of the White Paper was seen as postgraduate medical education and, particularly, medical audit (Downie & Charlton 1992). These have subsequently been observed to be slow and expensive. Purchasing authorities, if they employ the managerial regulation inherent within the contracting process, could achieve the same results more quickly and more directly (Charlton 1993). Should the development of the purchasing function therefore focus on the formulation of methodologies which would enable commissioners 'to stop purchasing activity and to begin purchasing evidence-based protocols' (Sheldon & Borowitz 1993)? Our opinion is firmly in the negative: it is simply too premature to do so. However, that a relationship exists between purchaser and provider in the promotion of quality in purchased and provided clinical practice is axiomatic. It is a question of the proper nature of that relationship relative to the likelihood of achieving the mutually desired end result.

Purchasing quality in clinical practice

In Chapter 1, Miles *et al.* examined the concept of *quality* in some detail, listing several definitions as part of their analysis. The definition by the Institute of Medicine that they recommend is of special relevance to the argument of this chapter, in terms of its aim in examining the relevance of the purchasing function in quality assurance and improvement within NHS provider organisations. The definition, which was synthesised by the Institute of Medicine after intensive research, is reiterated as:

'the degree to which health services for individuals and populations increase the likelihood of desired health outcomes and are consistent with current professional knowledge.'

(Lohr 1990; see also Palmer *et al.* 1991).

The utility of this definition in the context of this chapter is advanced as being manifest in three components:

(1) 'the degree to which ...' establishes the concept of variability which indicates the possibility of measurement, and thus quantification and qualitative description of the relevance of what has been quantified. It is therefore, as Wareham (1994a) has pointed out, singularly distinguished from a multiplicity of definitions which discuss quality in idealistic and absolute terms (Steffen 1988).

(2) 'the likelihood of desired outcomes' represents a frank recognition that outcomes may be anticipated but not guaranteed and that the relationship between process and outcome is probabilistic and not deterministic (Wareham 1994a).

(3) '... consistent with current knowledge' recognises the dependency of the standard of care on the status of scientific knowledge. It is in this context that we must consider what might be termed the objective status of scientific knowledge, that is the entire knowledge base which exists externally, to be referred to by any one clinician at any one time. This contrasts with the subjective status of scientific knowledge, that is the discrete body of knowledge possessed by an individual clinician; that highly variable quantity of scientific knowledge to which each individual clinician will refer in the treatment of each of his individual patients. Thus, while the standard of care is limited by the status and quantity of existing scientific knowledge and can thus be improved by each new contribution of clinical significance to the literature, it is limited especially and variably, by the status of knowledge of individual clinical practitioners. Hence the central utility of both undergraduate and continuing postgraduate education in ensuring the proper utilisation and assimilation of objectively existing knowledge and continuing medical advance.

Core ability of the purchasing function to influence the standard of care

Can the purchasing function *per se* increase the quality of care in a measurable and tangible manner by influencing the third of its three components: that care '... is consistent with current professional knowledge'? Some authors answer in the affirmative and proclaim the central utility of clinical practice guidelines in the healthcare purchasing process.

Donaldson (1994) has presented the process of healthcare purchasing with great diagrammatic clarity (Figure 8.1). It has been suggested that the consideration of guideline-based purchasing might take place at the first stage (establish what the population requires), a stage which Donaldson (1994) describes as:

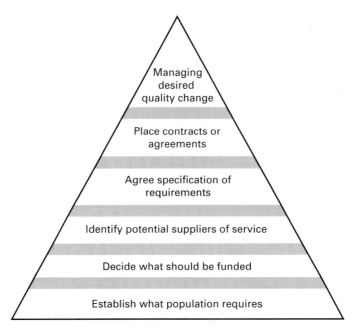

Fig. 8.1   The process of purchasing health care (Donaldson 1994). Reproduced with permission from BMJ Publishing Group.

'High quality management of the first step of the purchasing process would entail ensuring that the specification of the health care required by the population was based on sound epidemiological assessment of need, that it involved consumer perspectives, that it took account of the latest advances in medical knowledge and technology, and that comparisons were made with other services known to be doing better.

Purchasing highly specific packages of clinical care

Charlton (1993) predicted that purchasers would begin to consider this ideal and move increasingly towards a position of contracting for 'highly specific management packages', quoting guidance contained within *First Steps for the NHS* (NHSME 1992) and feared that 'what used to be decided at ground level by individual doctors will now be a contractual requirement'. But to what extent have the predictions of Charlton (1993) materialised to date? The contracting process is now relatively mature and, many authors had hoped that, by this time, purchasers would

'spend as much time successfully challenging ineffective or inappropriately accessed clinical practices as trying to contract within budget'.

(Gill 1993.)

In reality, progress has been slow and nervous, despite exhortations from protagonists of guideline-based healthcare commissioning.

Sheldon & Borowitz (1993) have advanced the contention that

> 'a key to improving quality in the NHS is for healthcare commissioners to stop purchasing activity and to begin purchasing evidence-based protocols'.

The authors base their contention on the reasoning that

> 'purchasing procedures or even packages of care guarantees nothing about the expected content and scientific basis of those services, whereas when a protocol is purchased we know that, if it is followed, the most effective set of actions will be taken'.

On first examination, how could such a contention be disputed? Who, for example, would doubt the therapeutic principle that purchasing authorities should: 'support and stimulate the development of guidelines and policies' (NHSME 1992) for thrombolytic treatment of acute myocardial infarction, especially given the extraordinary delay between the demonstration by cumulative meta-analysis of randomised controlled trials of the effectiveness of thrombolytic therapy in the preservation of left ventricular function following myocardial infarction and the initial introduction of this therapy into routine clinical practice (ISIS-2 1988; Collins & Julian 1991; Antman *et al.* 1992)? Indeed, there is evidence to suggest that the uptake may still not be as widespread as is acknowledged to be necessary (Ketley & Woods 1993; Lincolnshire MAAG 1994) and that ageism exists in its use (Dudley & Burns 1992). Should purchasing authorities – who are, after all, responsible for purchasing of services to meet epidemiologically indicated health need – not require, indeed mandate through financial prowess, that provider organisations must ensure that 100% of patients admitted with a diagnosis of acute myocardial infarction will, on the basis of ECG-indicated eligibility, receive thrombolysis within 25 minutes of arrival in the Accident & Emergency Department?

We must again reiterate our conclusion: no. Attempts to alter clinical practice in provider organisations through use of the contracting process are entirely unevaluated and potentially dangerous. The inclusion in health contracts of such mandates would certainly represent a discipline to clinicians, shifting the 'onus of proof', so that divergence from established protocols would require automatic justification by the clinician. However, poorly developed clinical guidelines can be misleading, confusing and can lead to inappropriate care (Gabbay & Stevens 1994). Donaldson (1994) felt that the health contract should not develop into a mechanism through which the purchasing authority could specify detailed procedures to the point where it becomes an operational manager by any other name, thus undermining the philosophy of the purchaser–provider split which required a devolution of operational issues to the level of the provider organisation. Charlton (1993) recognised that such measures would encourage reflective practice in clinicians and promote their use of 'scientific thinking' (Feinstein 1967; 1994), but warned of the creation of a dangerous precedent. Charlton suggested that the concept itself demonstrated a failure to recognise how science works and how medicine will best incorporate scientific advance into routine clinical practice.

External manipulation of clinical practice is unevaluated and potentially dangerous

It is for clinicians to direct such initiatives. Donaldson (1994) notes the anecdotes of contracts being agreed without involvement of medical staff and views it essential that the

> 'process of purchasing involves and gains the commitment of the senior professional staff who will actually be delivering the service'.

Initiatives aimed at guideline-based purchasing must involve and take advice from senior practitioners. There is clearly no benefit to be gained from requiring through contracts something which simply cannot in practice be delivered. To do so would be to place the purchaser and provider out of alignment and would lead to such initiatives being considered as 'foreign irritant(s) to be neutralised or repudiated' (Donabedian 1988). In taking the initiative, clinicians will preclude direction of their practice by non-clinical authorities who will certainly aim to institute practice changes under conditions where it has been judged that insufficient progress has been made by clinical professionals. Politicians, after all, believe that clinical guidelines are excellent mechanisms for introducing knowledge into practice and for reducing the gross costs of healthcare delivery (Secretary of State 1993) and are thus powerfully motivated in forcing guideline-directed change into routine operational practice. Medical development of this nature – where it is indicated necessary by definitive research evidence – is essential, but must resist dangerous interference and continue to occur in a 'bottom-up' manner. If it does not,

> 'responsibility for clinical standards would (pass) from the medical profession to the managerial structure – a change of direction with profound implications'.

(Charlton 1993.)

Clinical colleagues are divided, and not equally so, in the reception that they have afforded to the principle of the clinical guideline and the motivation that they have ascribed to the government in its promotion of the effectiveness initiative. A key political methodology for precipitating change in areas of known acute sensitivity within the medical profession is an incremental introduction of given policies so that individual changes, initially on a minor scale of significance, eventually act in concert to achieve the preconceived end result. This is simplistic, not very clever, but often highly effective. Thus, the initial proposals for guideline-based care emphasised the need to ensure clinically effective care, with little reference to cost. More recent directives have, however, increased the 'consciousness' of cost to a level where evidence of cost effectiveness is almost required to describe the clinical utility of given approaches to patient management. The appeal of a mechanism which would increase effectiveness at reduced cost is greater than one which will increase effectiveness at equal cost and is certainly infinitely more politically appealing than practice changes which will increase effectiveness at increased cost, no matter how great the increase in effectiveness might be.

Limitation of the standard of care by cost

The limitation of the standard of care by the objective and subjective status of clinical knowledge (see above) is itself augmented by the limitations imposed by the costs of care. As Donabedian *et al.* (1982) have pointed out, both individual and societal preferences directly influence the quality of care. Such factors have the capacity to produce sub-optimal care because of the opportunity costs involved in producing health care of 'higher quality'. This, as Wareham (1994a) has said, necessitates 'a political trade-off between cost and quality'. The same author argues that the consideration of cost in association with consideration of quality (Palmer *et al.* 1991) can act to focus attention on 'cost-containment rather than quality improvement'. It is certainly true that the lack of clarity between cost and quality generates conceptual and practical difficulties not uniquely experienced within the UK.

Drummond (1995), writing in the *Journal of Evaluation in Clinical Practice*, discusses the exponential growth in the publication of economic evaluations of healthcare treatments and programmes, citing two recent bibliographies (Backhouse *et al.* 1992: Elixhauser *et al.* 1993). These examples list in excess of 1000 works and augment the 150 studies described in the *Register of Cost-Effectiveness Studies* (DoH 1994). Indeed, Drummond (1994) is explicit in correlating the growth of and interest in such literature with the limitations on healthcare budgets. Interest shown by policy makers in a given area of research often reveals in advance the nature of subsequent policy. While there is currently limited evidence of economic data being used in the determination of clinical policy and its effects on healthcare delivery (Drummond 1995), it has been formally recommended that the protagonists and pioneers of 'evidence-based medicine' 'ought to embrace cost-effectiveness evidence as well as clinical evidence' (Drummond 1995). This author is clear, however, that the practice of including economic evaluation in clinical guideline and clinical policy formulation, for example economic analysis conducted in parallel with clinical trials, is a 'relatively young science'. It is nevertheless an innovation of which clinicians are understandably cautious and one viewed with no small suspicion.

Explicit consideration of cost continues to precipitate ethical and moral dilemmas among clinical colleagues. After all, clinicians have historically been trained to believe that they should provide ideal, rather than simply reasonable care to the people thay they have identified as needing it (Buchan 1993). Clearly, however, there is a need to include economic thinking in guideline development, if only to ensure that practices which result in large increases in cost for little increases in health gain, are avoided (Grimshaw *et al.* 1995b).

Many clinicians would entirely reject the suggestion that a given patient should be denied directly indicated care because of its cost. So how is the clinician to respond to the inexorably increasing pressure to act as 'bedside economist' as well as healer? How will he reconcile his professional obligation to deliver the 'best possible care' in situations where the best possible care, as defined clinically, is not affordable care as defined politically? Drummond (1995) argues that such sensitivities can be usefully addressed by health economics. This author points out that activities aimed at substituting high cost therapies with others demonstrated by clinical trials to be equivalent in effectiveness, are less exciting for clinicians than those activities directly targeted at improving the quality of patient care. He points out that such sub-stitutions can liberate resources that may enable new, more effective technologies to be employed. Drummond (1995) delineates some simple methodologies which enable the reality of resource constraint to be integrated into clinical decision-making. They are:

- decisions with specific reference to which drugs should be selected for inclusion in the formulary
- decisions with specific reference to the indications for use of particular drugs
- decisions with specific reference to the type of diagnostic workup given for particular kinds of patients
- decisions with specific reference to the patient risk factors that may indicate more or less intensive therapy.

When decisions are made, policy can be formulated, and formulated policy can be translated into practice guidelines. Such guidelines, when adopted locally, can result in local resource conservation, and when adopted nationally the extent of conservation can be of considerable significance.

It is therefore not surprising that political attention is focused pre-eminently on clinical guidelines. The introduction of the audit pro-gramme focused attention on the nature of professional practice (Secretaries of State for Health UK 1989), representing a tool with which excellence could be demonstrated, but also variation and eccentricity exposed. The research and development (R&D) pro-gramme has been aimed at facilitating the introduction of research evidence into routine clinical practice and stimulating the adoption of effective approaches to healthcare delivery (Peckham 1993). It is equally unsurprising to see that a particular synergy exists between both initiatives. Audit, in asking 'are we doing what we say we are?' is logically informed by R&D which asks 'what should we be doing?'

and, in an ideal situation, audit provides a definitive answer to such a question. A central difficulty is that definitive evidence for 'best clinical practice' is available in relatively few areas of a vast clinical art (Tanenbaum 1995). Clinicians are often distrustful of external recommendations, especially when contradictions are apparent, when multiple guidelines are recommended by different authorities for the same condition, where recommendations may be at odds with personal clinical experience and where legal responsibility, after all, remains firmly associated with individual clinical practice and individual clinical decision making. However, political pressure can be difficult to resist, especially when it is continuously and incrementally applied. It is in this context that we believe Charlton (1993) to have issued a salutary warning:

> 'Guidelines may stimulate thought in some clinicians but they will inhibit thought in others, who see little point in arguing with orders from above. Instead of doctors being educated to be autonomous practitioners of medical science, judgement will be taken from them. They would become passive functionaries following procedures devised by the great and good. Responsibility for clinical standards would have passed from the medical profession to the managerial structure – a change of direction with profound implications.'

Guideline-based, purchaser-driven care: the extent of progress to date

The indications are, however, that the process of purchasing protocols of care has progressed slowly, despite communications from the NHS Executive urging purchasers, GP fundholders and Trusts to take account of clinical effectiveness and clinical guidelines in the contracting process (NHS Executive 1993) and guidance for 1995/6 planning emphasised the importance of investing

> 'an increasing proportion of resources in interventions known to be effective and where outcomes can be systematically monitored'.
> (NHSME 1994b.)

A reduction in 'investment in interventions shown to be less effective' was to accompany this process. Purchasing authorities were expected to demonstrate their consideration of this guidance by increasing their investment in two interventions known to be effective and to reduce their investment in two interventions demonstrated by effectiveness research to be essentially ineffective. In addition, purchasing authorities were required to promote a greater use of the clinical audit process in health contracts.

Further guidance in the same year clarified objectives and recognised the complexity of the process and the investment of time that was required to modify clinical guidelines for use in local health settings (NHSME 1994c). As Hayward (1994) has said, this 'softening of approach' was welcome, especially given the evidence demonstrating that a 'top-down' approach (Charlton 1993) was unlikely to change behaviour as effectively as local clinicians developing local guidelines (Grimshaw & Russell 1993a). A comprehensive collaboration in this context was recommended by the guidance through the involvement of clinicians and agencies in the primary healthcare setting, and one which should not exclude consultation with patients (see Chapter 11).

Ham *et al.* (1995) have emphasised that policy making within the health service should, like clinical care, be evidence based. On what evidence, then, has the policy for purchasing protocols of care been based? There is no evidence to demonstrate that the purchasing mechanism can achieve completely rational, systematic and evidence-based healthcare in provider organisations. Instead, advocates of this policy adopt an assumptive and theoretical approach which fails to demonstrate that it has considered the principal difficulties involved in implementing such a policy in hard, operational terms. Real breakthoughs, as Charlton (1993) has pointed out, are rare, and the derivation of the medical evidence, like those who judge it appropriate for immediate introduction into routine clinical practice, needs to be scrutinised exactingly. Much of what has been written appears to have failed to take into account the complexity of the clinical decision-making process at the level of the individual patient. Miles (1995a, b) has emphasised the uncertainty of the limits to which general research evidence can be applied to individual patients and many clinicians would agree that

> 'clinical and moral knowledge of individual patients is subjective and implicit and this will remain the case no matter how many clinical trials are performed'.
>
> (Feder 1994a.)

Naylor (1995), for example, is clear in pointing out that

> 'clinical medicine seems to consist of a few things we know, a few things we think we know, but probably don't, and lots of things we don't know at all'.

Many clinical actions cannot be guided by evidence alone: definitive evidence will often not exist, clinicians may be unsatisfied as to its integrity and it may simply be inapplicable to a given individual patient. As a consequence, many clinicians become skilled in 'educated guesswork' and in many clinical situations it is more a question of 'reconciling the new evaluative sciences and old arts' than mandating the use of clinical guidelines which may have 'failed to distinguish fact from fervour' (Naylor 1995). Rigge, in outlining the patient's view of guidelines in Chapter 11, is clear:

> 'the very term "guidelines" suggests ... that they are something you steer by ... it is clearly in everyone's interest to encourage the

development of evidence-based medicine, but this must be done in the context both of medical and scientific uncertainty and of the uniqueness of every transaction that takes place between doctors and their patients'.

Hayward (1994) was clear that the use of the contracting mechanism to change clinical practice within provider units would be 'mechanistic' at the present time and requires evaluation. This author believed that purchasers should have a more interactive role, establishing dialogue with local hospital doctors, GPs and patients, and insisting that hospital doctors address policy and practice in light of the research evidence that is increasingly being made available by the Cochrane Collaboration and the NHS Centre for Reviews and Dissemination. Hayward (1994) suggests that the role of the contracting mechanism in the effectiveness movement may be manifest in ensuring that productive dialogue takes place between these groups. Miles *et al.* in Chapters 3 and 4 have advanced a mechanism through which such dialogue can be maintained in operational practice.

Biting the bullet or inviting one? Definitive decision making in the purchasing process

A simplistic approach to purchasing healthcare through guidelines may also precipitate moral, ethical and medico-legal difficulties. As Drummond (1995) concedes, 'few therapies are completely worthless. Usually the question is one of how much they should be used'. What, for example, could health commissioners stop purchasing? Gastric freezing? Extracranial–intracranial bypass? Dilation and curettage in young women? Surgery for glue ear? Tubal surgery in women with moderate to severe obstruction (Beeson 1980: Effective Health Care Bulletin 1992a, b; Coulter *et al.* 1993)? While some interventions are recognised to be definitively ineffective, for example, gastric freezing (Beeson 1980), the effectiveness of others will depend on multiple factors. It is recognised that surgery for glue ear is in many cases valueless (and is likely to be ineffective if the hearing loss is less than 25dB), yet some children with lower levels of hearing loss have been shown to benefit (Black *et al.* 1990). Prostatectomy is similarly considered to be ineffective in relieving mild symptoms compared to severe symptoms but research has shown that some men with mild symptoms can show clinical improvement (Flood *et al.* 1992).

Purchasing decisions could also, theoretically at least, be taken when clinical interventions or diagnostic techniques are of equal effectiveness but differing cost, when less effective clinical interventions are more expensive or where relatively small numbers of given clinical procedures are performed in a given provider organisation, a situation associated with poor clinical outcome (Luft 1980; Song *et al.* 1993; McKee & Clarke 1995). In Chapter 7 of this volume, Bentley *et al.* suggest that cosmetic operations may be deliberately excluded from the range of services purchased without any reduction in the health of the population. In Chapter 5, Haines *et al.* contend that

> 'if it were desired to prevent the use of an inappropriate surgical procedure, the commissioning process might be an effective lever in that commissioners could exclude such procedures from contracts'.

The theory of this approach is all very well, but what is inappropriate and what is not within highly varying patient populations? Furthermore, what is the nature and weight of evidence which would be employed in such decision making? We believe that such questions raise the matter of competence to judge.

Competence to judge: necessity for a central, authoritative professional body in developing guideline-driven care

Charlton (1993) is clear in rejecting the identification of 'clinically important facts' by NHS Management Executive-appointed expert panels as 'science', viewing it as a 'top-down' autocratic process that is diametrically opposed to the 'bottom-up' democratic process of science. This author feels that establishing a managerial influence over the implementation of research may well result in science being defined using politically expedient criteria, thereby not representing science at all. The use of politically acceptable, rather than scientifically valid practices, may result.

Data on the integrity of clinical guidelines is vital if clinicians are to be persuaded to adopt them, but how – in the face of proliferating local (Littlejohns & Sharda 1994) and national (Feder 1994a, b) guidelines – are clinicians to be persuaded of guideline integrity, and how will purchasers achieve the managerial (and legal) confidence strongly to encourage their use through the purchasing mechanism? In an important work, Cluzeau *et al.* (1994) considered the potential utility of a *Which?* style guide through which clinicians and managers in their respective settings and from their respective viewpoints, might agree on local approaches to healthcare provision. The authors argued that a principal characteristic of such a *Which?* guide would be its ability to identify 'valid' guidelines, that is guidelines which had been appraised against predefined criteria. More specifically, the guide would recommend a guideline only if adherence to it would 'increase the probability of bringing about the expected health outcome at the expected cost' (Cluzeau *et al.* 1994).

It is immediately clear that a great deal of data is necessary to judge validity in this context and it is well acknowledged that the majority of clinical guidelines available currently have not been published with clear reference to the data and methodology employed in their derivation (Grimshaw & Russell 1993b; Grimshaw 1994; Grimshaw *et al.* 1995a, b). A further complexity is represented by the issue of competence to judge. No organisational framework currently exists to undertake such an exercise and local attempts to do so by purchasers and providers will lead, as Cluzeau *et al.* (1994) have suggested, to duplication of efforts and diseconomies of small scale. A co-ordination of national professional bodies would appear to be fundamental to achieving 'competence to judge' and in conferring authority on such a *Which?* guide. There is evidence that guideline development is now beginning to proceed more rigorously and with greater reference to pre-existing understanding (Field & Lohr 1992) as well as to developed understanding (Grimshaw *et al.* 1995a, b). Until the guidelines produced in this revised manner have been rigorously scrutinised by competent professional authority, the introduction of a national *Which?* guide, or the development of a local one, remains 'premature' (Cluzeau *et al.* 1994).

Adherence to clinical guidelines within NHS provider units: the utility of internal and external monitoring mechanisms

How will purchasing authorities – in circumstances where guidelines based on definitive, clinically accepted evidence are being purchased – satisfy themselves that the care provided in their commissioned provider organisations meets given standards and is therefore satisfactory? The concern for meeting standards is shared by the provider organisations themselves. Clinicians must meet standards for noble, Hippocratic reasons, while managers must ensure that they are in a position to report that this has been the case, to maintain (and potentially increase) contracted activity and its associated resourcing. The answer is likely to lie in the establishment of internal and external systems of monitoring. But what form will these take?

Purchasers may need to consider considerable investment in what some authors have termed 'quality police' (Boufford 1993; McKee & Clarke 1995), administrative officers who would be required to maintain a largely *external monitoring* of adherence to clinical standards and guidelines. NHS management numbers and costs are increased in this way, with economic and political complications. Indeed, Boufford (1993) feels certain that purchasing authorities will never be in a position to appoint the necessary number of staff for adequate monitoring of general quality initiatives of which guideline implementation will represent a prominent activity. Monitoring adherence to clinical guidelines is a complex procedure requiring particular skills and a great deal of time, as Chapters 3 and 4 have described. It also assumes that clinicians will comply in corporate fashion with guideline-based purchaser-driven healthcare delivery. Such corporate acceptance does not yet characterise the general disposition of clinicians in this context.

External monitoring

External quality monitoring is, by definition, conducted by organisations that are external and from which an objective assessment may be anticipated, but not necessarily guaranteed. Purchasing authorities may have their own particular agenda in dealing with their provider organisations, especially those which have experienced difficulty in implementing a functional purchaser–provider split and continue to behave in the manner of the old district health authorities.

Internal monitoring

External monitoring is immediately distinguished from internal quality review which, as its description suggests, is conducted internally by the provider organisation itself. An objective assessment may be anticipated on the grounds of integrity though, again, cannot be guaranteed, and there may be selection in what is studied and in what is reported when the study of a given area of care has been completed. Why should such selection occur? The answer is simple (and though not palatable, quite possible): the NHS now conducts its business in the market place and in the market place there is competition. Where there is competition there is commercial sensitivity. Where there is commercial sensitivity, pragmatic approaches are adopted to deal with it. A mechanism is therefore required to ensure objectivity of observation and interpretation by both purchasers and providers.

Optimum methodologies for monitoring

Wareham (1994a) believes that internal and external quality monitoring are 'distinct concepts that in reality cannot exist as entirely separate entities' and it is argued that approaches to their consideration as alternatives can lead to the 'polarisation of two mechanisms which are inherently symbiotic' (Berwick 1990; 1992; Wareham 1994a). Wareham (1994b) is succinct in this context:

> 'A global system of quality improvement based solely on internal quality improvement presents insurmountable problems as it would be devoid of a system of public protection and external accountability. Conversely, an entirely external system would be equally insupportable because it would have to rely entirely on inspection, generating a cycle of fear and antagonism and would not create an environment likely to support improvement.'

We believe that a system of external review complements internal review, assists it, confirms its results and is highly desirable within a competitive marketplace.

Central utility of audit data in purchasing quality in clinical care

Audit data are central to the monitoring of clinical quality. Since it is our contention that clinical quality may be assessed in terms of the effectiveness and appropriateness of clinical intervention, and also in terms of the efficiency with which effective, appropriate care is delivered to patients, we believe that audit programmes and methodologies must focus on examination and measurement of effectiveness, appropriateness and efficiency. Purchasers are increasingly concerned to set the parameters for clinical audit programmes. Indeed, as O'Neill pointed out in Chapter 6, purchaser concerns may now – on the basis of guidance from the NHS Executive – constitute 40% of local provider audit agendas. Haines *et al.* (Chapter 5) view this as an opportunity for purchasers to be 'well placed to ensure that clinical effectiveness in specific fields is monitored'. Such monitoring, examination and measurement may be conducted as part of internal quality review and may be confirmed by external review. This process may involve a statistically valid sampling of provider supplied results and their subsequent verification by repeat analysis. That is, the testing for discrepancy between what is found by the purchaser and what has been reported by the provider in the same patient cases. For such an exercise it is clearly essential that medical record numbers and raw data are retained as part of every audit so that such direct discrepancy testing can be performed and any differences identified, discussed and explained. Such an exercise can be performed easily by purchasers, is essentially constructive and does not necessitate an 'army of quality police' (Boufford 1993; McKee & Clarke 1995).

Quantitative assessment of the nature and extent of guideline implementation in NHS provider organisations

Chapters 3 and 4 of this volume presented a system for evaluating the totality of clinical care which describes a method through which purchasers may achieve effective monitoring in operational practice. Specifically, the method facilitates the comparison and contrast of existing local practice with evidence-based practice, promotes the agreement of change aimed at narrowing the discrepancy between the two and specifically enables the nature and extent of implementation of that change to be precisely assessed. The reader is therefore referred to those sections for more detailed discussion.

Objections of clinical staff to external monitoring of quality in clinical practice

Roche (1994) has pointed out that

'many clinicians would be reluctant to release audit results at the point where a problem had been identified, but would be willing to share the results of the completed projects, after remedial action has been taken and a change in practice demonstrated'.

Many investigators do not share Roche's confidence that remedial action and change in practice follow *ipso facto* from identification of deficiency and a role of purchasers in facilitating this process, though mutual discussion of so-called 'bad' audit results can facilitate continuous quality improvement. Indeed, as Thomson (1994) has said, purchasers should ask '*Can* this hospital provide good quality care?' and not simply '*Does* this hospital produce good quality care?'. Such an approach is powerful in precluding the view of the purchaser as 'a foreign irritant to be neutralised or repudiated' (Donabedian 1988) and Miles *et al.* (Chapters 3 and 4) have argued emphatically for a functional role of the purchaser in the executive management and interpretation of provider audit.

Access of commissioners to provider audit results

If audit data of the nature described in Chapters 3 and 4 are accepted as of central value in the external and internal monitoring process, it follows that commissioners must begin to adopt serious approaches to the development of monitoring mechanisms that show complementarity and compatibility with systems of provider audit and internal monitoring activities. The success of the purchaser–provider relationship will be dependent in large measure on the ability of each to be sure of the other's competence within the exercise of their established remits (that is, purchasing and providing). This emphasises, rather singularly, the need for intimate collaboration and adds force to the arguments expressed in Chapters 3 and 4 for a functional role of the purchaser in the entire process of provider continuous clinical quality improvement.

But how effective is the purchaser in gaining access to, interpreting and basing managerial decisions on audit results? A comprehensive study of purchasing authorities' involvement in audit was undertaken by Rumsey *et al.* (1994) which largely confirmed the view that the use of the audit process and its results in the purchasing function is spectacularly under-developed. Rumsey *et al.* examined the characteristics of purchaser involvement in provider audit in 86 of 123 purchasing authorites identified in England, observing the involvement of purchasers to be largely 'reactive and paper-based' and relying substantially on the receipt of written reports from their provider organisations. Commissioners expressed a general dissatisfaction with the 'quality and completeness' of submitted audit reports and, in approximately half of cases studied, commissioning authorities did not consider that the reports they received helped identify any real quality improvements in the general service delivery. The receipt of retrospective information only was a prominent feature of the reports received by purchasing authorities which, as Rumsey pointed out, probably acts to limit the ability of the commissioning function to influence the direction of audit in local provider organisations. It is gratifying to note, however, that the purchasing authorities investigated expressed definitive interest in the receipt of improved audit reports and in precise details of the nature and extent of quality improvements resulting from provider audit. It is now timely that such definitive interest is translated into definitive action and, for our part, we recommend the methodological approach described above as an essential component of any strategy being formulated for development of the purchaser function.

Need to develop academically tenable methodologies

Patience is necessary in the development of the methodologies necessary to support the development of adequate monitoring mechanisms and it must be recognised that

> 'compromises between political expectations of immediate impact and an academic need for a considered development of measurement methods'
>
> (Wareham 1994a)

result, in our view, in a compromised validity and therefore utility of the whole process. They therefore frustrate the achievement of the mutually desired end-result.

Paucity of examples of effective internal and external monitoring

Wareham (1994b) has pointed out that there are, as yet, no splendid examples of systems which have perfected a complementary, compatible mix of internal and external monitoring mechanisms. Those who are given responsibility for designing successful methodologies face difficult tasks in formulating methodologies which will secure a functional integration between internal and external quality monitoring systems (Vladeck 1988; Berwick 1990; 1992; Merry 1991; Roberts 1991; Brooks *et al.* 1992; US General Accounting Office 1992).

Conclusion

Scrutiny of the purchasing mechanism – as it exists at the time of writing – demonstrates the limitations of its ability to precipitate changes in clinical practice within provider organisations. There are extensive areas in medicine where purchasing-guideline based care will prove extremely difficult if not impossible, but there are many areas amenable to external influences derived from evidence-based medicine and evidence-based policy. This does not obviate, but rather underlines, the need for further research, further education and further stimulation of local guideline development, all of which can be markedly promoted, not forced, through health contracts. Such an approach is likely to show wisdom, rather than the opposite and will demonstrate that purchasing authorities have a firm belief in the maxim: 'more haste, less speed'.

References

Antman, E., Lau, J., Kupelnick, B., Mosteller, F. & Chalmers, I. (1992) A comparison of the results of meta-analysis of randomised controlled trials and recommendations of clinical experts. *Journal of the American Medical Association* **268**: 240–48.

Backhouse, M.E., Backhouse, R.J. & Edey, S.A. (1992) Economic evaluation bibliography. *Health Economics* **1** (Suppl.): 1–236.

Beecham, L. (1994) Tories extend general practice fundholding. *British Medical Journal* **309**: 1039.

Beeson, P. (1980) Changes in medical therapy. *Medicine* **59**: 79–84.

Berwick, D.M. (1990) Peer-review and quality management: are they compatible? *Quarterly Review Bulletin* **16**: 46–51.

Berwick, D.M. (1992) Heal thyself or heal the system: can doctors help to improve medical care? *Quality in Health Care* **1** (Suppl.): 2–8.

Black, N.A., Sanderson, C.F., Freeland, A.M. & Vessey, P.M. (1990) A randomised controlled trial of surgery for glue ear. *British Medical Journal* **300**: 1551–6.

Boufford, J.L. (1993) US and UK health care reforms: reflections on quality. *Quality in Health Care* **2**: 249–52.

Brooks, J.H.J., Renz, K.K. & Richardson, S.L. (1992) Systems versus performance problems: a peer-review organisation's perspective. *Quarterly Review Bulletin* **18**: 172–7.

Buchan, H. (1993) Clinical guidelines: acceptance and promotion. *Quality in Health Care* **2**: 213–14.

Bunker, J. (1994) Can professionalism survive in the marketplace? *British Medical Journal* **308**: 1179–80.

Charlton, B.G. (1993) Management of science. *Lancet* **342**: 99–100.

Cluzeau, F., Littlejohns, P. & Grimshaw, J.M. (1994) Appraising clinical guidelines: towards a *Which?* guide for purchasers. *Quality in Health Care* **3**: 121–2.

Collins, R. & Julian, D. (1991) British Heart Foundation surveys (1987 and 1989) of United Kingdom treatment policies for acute myocardial infarction. *British Heart Journal* **66**: 2505.

Coulter, A., Klassen, A., MacKenzie, I.Z. & McPherson, K. (1993) Diagnostic dilation and curettage – is it used appropriately? *British Medical Journal* **306**: 236–9.

DoH (1994) *Register of Cost-Effectiveness Studies*, Department of Health, HMSO, London.

Donabedian, A. (1988) Quality assessment and assurance: unity of purpose, diversity of means. *Inquiry* **25**: 173–92.

Donabedian, A., Wheeler, J.R.C. & Wyszewianski, L. (1982) Quality, cost and health: an integrative model. *Medical Care* **20**: 975–92.

Donaldson, L. (1994) Building quality into contracting and purchasing. *Quality in Health Care* **3** (Suppl.): S37–S40.

Downie, R.S. & Charlton, B. (1992) *The Making of a Doctor: Medical Education in Theory and Practice*, Oxford University Press, Oxford.

Drummond, M. (1994) *Economic Analysis Alongside Controlled Trials: An Introduction For Clinical Researchers*, Department of Health, HMSO; London.

Drummond, M. (1995) The role of health economics in clinical evaluation. *Journal of Evaluation in Clinical Practice* **1**: 71–5.

Dudley, N.J. & Burns, E. (1992) The influence of age on policies for admission and thrombolysis in coronary care units in the United Kingdom. *Age and Ageing* **21**: 95–8.

Effective Health Care Bulletin (1992a) *The Management of Persistent Glue Ear in Children*, University of Leeds, Leeds.

Effective Health Care Bulletin (1992b) *Management of Infertility*, University of Leeds, Leeds.

Elixhauser, A., Luce, B.R., Taylor, W.R. & Reblando, J. (1993) Health care CBA/ CEA: an update on the growth and composition of the literature. *Medical Care* **31** (Suppl.): JS1–JS11.

Feder, G. (1994a) Clinical guidelines in 1994. *British Medical Journal* **309**: 1457–8.

Feder, G. (1994b) Which guidelines to follow? *British Medical Journal* **305**: 785–6.

Feinstein, A.R. (1967) *Clinical Judgement*, Williams and Wilkins, Baltimore, MD.

Feinstein, A.R. (1994) Clinical judgement revisited – the distraction of quantitative models. *Annals of Internal Medicine* **120**: 799–805.

Field, M.J. & Lohr, K. (1992) *Guidelines for Clinical Practice: From Development to Use*, National Academy Press, Washington, DC.

Flood, A.B., Black, N.A., McPherson, K., Smith, J. & Williams, G. (1992) Assessing symptom improvement after elective prostatectomy for benign prostatic hypertrophy. *Archives of Internal Medicine* **152**: 1507–12.

Gabbay, J. & Stevens, A. (1994) Towards investing in health gain. *British Medical Journal* **308**: 1117–18.

Gill, M. (1993) Purchasing for quality: still in the starting blocks? *Quality in Health Care* **2**: 179–82.

Grimshaw, J.M. (1994) Guidelines. *British Medical Journal* **307**: 1531.

Grimshaw, J.M. & Russell, I. (1993a) Effect of clinical guidelines on medical practice: a systematic review of rigorous evaluations. *Lancet* **342**: 1317–22.

Grimshaw, J.M. & Russell, I. (1993b) Achieving health gain through clinical guidelines I. Developing scientifically valid guidelines. *Quality in Health Care* **2**: 243–8.

Grimshaw, J.M., Eccles, M. and Russell, I.T. (1995a) Developing clinically valid practice guidelines. *Journal of Evaluation in Clinical Practice* **1**: 37–48.

Grimshaw, J.M., Freemantle, N., Wallace, S., Russell, I., Hurwitz, B., Watt, I., Long, A. & Sheldon, T. (1995b) Developing and implementing clinical practice guidelines. *Quality in Health Care* **4**: 55–64.

Ham, C. (1994) The future of purchasing – tolerance of diversity will be necessary. *British Medical Journal* **309**: 1032–3.

Ham, C., Hunter, D. & Robinson, R. (1995) Evidence-based policy-making: research must inform health policy as well as medical care. *British Medical Journal* **310**: 71–2.

Hayward, J. (1994) Purchasing clinically effective care. *British Medical Journal* **309**: 823–5.

ISIS-2 (1988) Second International Study of Infarct Survival. Randomised trial of intravenous steptokinase, oral aspirin, both or neither among 17 187 cases of suspected acute myocardial infarction. *Lancet* **ii**: 349–60.

Ketley, D. & Woods, K.L. (1993) Impact of clinical trials on clinical practice: example of thrombolysis for acute myocardial infarction. *Lancet* **342**: 891–4.

Kirkup, B. & Donaldson, L.J. (1994) Is healthcare a commodity: how will purchasing improve the NHS? *Journal of Public Health Medicine* **16**: 256–62.

Komaroff, A.L. (1978) The PRSO, quality assurance blues. *New England Journal of Medicine* **298**: 1194–6.

Lincolnshire MAAG (1994) *Audit of Management of Suspected Heart Attacks*, Lincolnshire Medical Audit Advisory Group, Lincoln.

Littlejohns, P. & Sharda, A. (1994) Guidelines and protocols for sharing of health care between hospitals and general practitioners in south west Thames. *Medical Audit News* **4**: 1–2.

Lohr, K. (1990) *Medicare: A Strategy for Quality Assurance*, Institute of Medicine, National Academy Press, Washington, DC.

Loughlin, M. (1993) The illusion of quality. *Health Care Analysis* **1**: 69–73.

Loughlin, M. (1994) The poverty of management. *Health Care Analysis* **2**: 135–9.

Loughlin, M. (1995) Brief encounter: a dialogue between a philosopher and an NHS manager on the subject of 'quality'. *Journal of Evaluation in Clinical Practice* **1**: 81–5.

Luft, H.S. (1980) The relationship between surgical volume and mortality: an exploration of causal factors and alternative models. *Medical Care* **18**: 940–59.

Maynard, A. (1993) Never mind the quality? *Health Service Journal*, 11 March: 21.

McKee, M. & Clarke, A. (1995) Guidelines, enthusiasm, uncertainty and the limits to purchasing. *British Medical Journal* **310**: 101–104.

Merry, M.D. (1991) Can an external review system avoid the inspection model? *Quarterly Review Bulletin* **17**: 315–19.

Miles, A. (1995a) Critical inquiry into clinical practice. *Journal of Evaluation in Clinical Practice* **1**: 3–4.

Miles, A. (1995b) Purchasing quality in clinical practice: what on earth do we mean? *Journal of Evaluation in Clinical Practice* **1**: 81–4.

Naylor, D.C. (1995) Grey zones of clinical practice: some limits to evidence-based medicine. *Lancet* **345**: 842–52.

NHSME (1992) *First Steps for the NHS*, NHS Management Executive, Department of Health, Leeds.

NHSME (1993) *Improving Clinical Effectiveness*, EL(93)115, NHS Executive, Department of Health, Leeds.

NHSME (1994a) *Developing NHS Purchasing and GP Fundholding*, EL(94)79, NHS Management Executive, Department of Health, Leeds.

NHSME (1994b) *Priorities and Planning Guidance for the NHS: 1995/1996*, EL(94)55, NHS Management Executive, Department of Health, Leeds.

NHSME (1994c) *Improving the Effectiveness of the NHS*, EL(94)74, NHS Management Executive, Department of Health, Leeds.

Palmer, R.H., Donabedian, A. & Pover, G.J. (1991) *Striving for Quality in Health Care: An Inquiry Into Policy and Practice*, Health Administration Press, Ann Arbor, MI.

Parmley, W.W. (1994). Clinical practice guidelines. Does the cookbook have enough recipes? *Journal of the American Medical Association* **272**: 1374–5.

Peckham, M. (1993) *Research for Health*, Department of Health, HMSO, London.

Roberts, J.S. (1991) External review in the brave new world of continuous quality improvement. *Quarterly Review Bulletin* **17**: 314.

Robinson, R. (1994) Evaluating the NHS reforms. In: *Evaluating the NHS Reforms*, (eds R. Robinson and J. Le Grand). King's Fund Institute, London.

Roche, M. (1994) Clinical audit and the purchaser. *Auditorium* **1**: 6–7.

Rothwell, P.M. (1995) Can overall results of clinical trials be applied to all patients? *Lancet* **345**: 1616–18.

Rumsey, M., Walshe, K., Bennett, J. & Coles, J. (1994) *The role of the Commissioner in Audit – Findings of a National Survey of Commissioning Authorities in England*, CASPE, London.

Secretaries of State for Health UK (1989) *Working for Patients*, CM555, HMSO, London.

Secretary of State (1993) Speech delivered to BMA/King's Fund/Patients' Association Conference, 11 March 1993. *Health Care Analysis* **2**: 5–12.

Shapiro, J. (1994) *Shared Purchasing and Collaborative Commissioning with the NHS*, National Association of Health Authorities and Trusts, Birmingham.

Sheldon, T. & Borowitz, M. (1993) Changing the measure of quality in the NHS: from purchasing activity to purchasing protocols. *Quality in Health Care* **2**: 149–50.

Song, F., Freemantle, N., Sheldon, T., House, A., Watson, P. & Long, A. (1993) Selective serotonin reuptake inhibitors: meta-analysis of efficacy and acceptability. *British Medical Journal* **306**: 683–7.

Steffen, G.E. (1988) Quality medical care: a definition. *Journal of the American Medical Association* **260**: 56–61.

Tanenbaum, S. (1995) Getting there from here: evidentiary quandaries of the US outcomes movement. *Journal of Evaluation in Clinical Practice* **1**: 97–103.

Thomson, R. (1994) The purchaser role in provider quality: lessons from the United States. *Quality in Health Care* **3**: 65–6.

US General Accounting Office (1990) *Quality Assurance: a Comprehensive National Strategy for Health Care is needed*. US General Accounting Office, Washington, DC.

US General Accounting Office (1992) *Utilisation Review: Information on External Review Organisations*, US General Accounting Office, Washington, DC.

Vladeck, B.C. (1988) Quality assurance through external controls. *Inquiry* **25**: 100–107.

Wareham, N.J. (1994a) External monitoring of quality of health care in the United States. *Quality in Health Care* **3**: 97–101.

Wareham, N.J. (1994b) Changing systems of external monitoring of quality of health care in the United States. *Quality in Health Care* **3**: 102–106.

Wennberg, J.E. (1990) Innovation and the policies of limits in a changing healthcare economy. In: *Modern Methods of Clinical Investigation*, (ed. A. Gelijns), pp. 9–33. National Academy Press, Washington, DC.

9 ◆ The Authority and Legal Standing of Clinical Standards and Practice Guidelines

Brian Hurwitz

'What usually is done may be evidence of what ought to be done ... but what ought to be done is fixed by a standard of reasonable prudence, whether it is complied with or not.'

(Holmes 1903.)

'[In] cases involving particular treatment decisions, the role of protocols and guidelines will become more and more significant in determining whether a doctor has violated the law.'

(Kennedy 1993.)

Introduction

In the 1994 legal case of *Early v. Newham Health Authority* it was alleged that an anaesthetist had employed a faulty protocol during a failed intubation procedure (*Early* 1994). A 13-year-old girl had awoken while still paralysed from suxemethonium. She charged that the protocol used in her care, which recommended insufflation of the lungs with an oxygen rich mixture rather than an oxygen and anaesthetic mixture, had caused avoidable injury. On regaining consciousness, she had suffered fright and distress as a result of the suxemethonium paralysis which had not worn off.

The judge heard evidence about the protocol's origin, its development and manner of adoption, and was informed of its use in other UK hospitals. Notwithstanding the testimony of a professor of anaesthesia when referring to the protocol, that: '... no reasonably competent medical authority would have condoned this drill', the judge found in favour of the defendants, observing that the authors of this particular protocol had been responsible and competent and that the health authority had not been negligent in approving it.

Proliferation of clinical standards, guidelines and protocols reflects important changes in the culture of the NHS. In discussing the place of modern healthcare in society, a distinguished professor of medical law has written:

'The sense of belonging to a flawed but noble enterprise where everyone gained a little bit, where the system tried to do its best for all by all, is going ... the language is now of consumers, providers,

purchasers, charters, enterprise, targets. Well, these changes in ethos
... in the notion of the NHS, will, I predict ... produce a sea change in
the role of recourse to law. [T]he law ... deals everyday with the
language of consumers, users, charters, purchasers and contracts.
This is the language of law, especially when coupled with accompanying rhetoric about rights.'

(Kennedy 1993.)

In the UK, proliferation of standards and guidelines also reflects a
change in the regulatory framework of healthcare, from one in which
professional stewardship once predominated, to one increasingly
influenced by quasi-market mechanisms and civil regulation. Viewed
as markers of quality which can be audited and taken account of in the
contracting process, the healthcare market is beginning to assign
standards and guidelines major roles in mediating the delivery of
healthcare (Ellman 1989; Healthcare Standards Directory 1993; Hopkins 1993). Where a healthcare market has long operated in the USA,
some 20 000 clinical standards and practice guidelines are reputedly in
circulation (Leone 1993), with the result that American physicians now
believe themselves to be 'pinioned by regulations and controls far
beyond ... colleagues in most other countries' (Silver 1987).

Doctors are not generally trained to recognise when a clinical
guideline represents mere guidance, and when it is an authoritative
recommendation. Understanding the nature of the authority (if any) of
advisory statements proclaiming to be standards or guidelines is
essential to the development of a mature professional response to their
appearance. *Early v Newham Health Authority* shows that compliance
with certain standards or protocols may not automatically protect
clinicians from liability if patients suffer harm during treatment.

Because the status and authority of clinical standards and guidelines
are variable and not always transparent (Cluzeau *et al.* 1994), protocols
and guidelines remain open to contest in court. This chapter examines
the different kinds of authority embodied in guideline documents, and
reviews the use which courts have made of these statements in
deciding cases alleging medical negligence.

What are standards and guidelines?

Standards

Essential to the notion of a 'standard' is that of reference, by which
some activity or object can be compared and judged. Samuel Johnson
said of standards generally that they were 'of undoubted authority',
'the test of other things' and had themselves been 'tried by the proper
test' (Chalmers, A. 1994). The *Oxford English Dictionary* defines 'standard' as 'a definite degree of excellence' and 'an authoritative or
recognised exemplar of correctness, perfection, or some definite degree
of quality'. The simultaneous co-existence of different standards for the
care of the same condition shows that though clinical standards may

abound, they may fail to provide reliable yardsticks for the purposes of clinical care (or research). Where consensus between different clinical standards seems close, its statement may still result in a composite of different recommendations of widely differing status (CSAGC 1994: 13).

Debate about how to develop standards and guidelines for clinical performance often centres on methodological (and philosophical) issues concerning how to devise 'proper tests' of clinical activity (Chalmers, I. 1994). Standards representing differing degrees of 'stringency' are required for different purposes: a useful hierarchy is provided by the US Institute of Medicine, which divides authoritative statements of clinical standards into:

'(1) minimum levels of acceptable performance or results,
(2) excellent levels of performance or results, or
(3) the range of acceptable performance or results'.

(Field & Lohr 1990.)

Guidelines

Although of obvious significance to doctors, clinical guidelines occupy but a small part of a wider discourse concerning how society chooses to regulate certain activities generally. In public affairs, guidelines are now held to govern the conduct of cabinet ministers, the sale of arms to foreign countries and the operation of professional parliamentary lobby groups. The term also features on packaged food labels, as reheating and cooking 'guidelines', and in the documentation sent by medical journals to aspiring contributors: 'guidelines for authors' (Anonymous 1991a), and 'guidelines for referees' (Anonymous 1991b). Applications of all sorts, whether for memberships or mortgages, are frequently accompanied by requests to adhere to 'guidelines' designed to ensure that application is made in a proper manner.

By analogy with a plumbline, guidelines have been invented (and distributed) in order to be followed. But unlike a plumbline, which is invariably governed by a reliable natural force and is therefore always authoritative in delineating a standard (the vertical), clinical protocols and guidelines are not identical with clinical standards. On the contrary, guidelines derive from authorities of widely varying reliability, embody goals originating from outside the immediate doctor–patient relationship, and may even seem at odds with the best interests of particular patients (Feder 1994; McKee & Clarke 1995).

For a term that finds application in areas as diverse as cooks and cabinet ministers, it is worth noting that 'guideline' lacks a distinctive dictionary definition, its meaning having been stretched 'to include too many different kinds of guidance' (McDonald & Overhage 1994). In a medical context, the term is frequently used loosely. 'Guidelines' increasingly appear where 'guidance', 'recommendation' or simply 'advice' previously sufficed. Consider Victoria Gillick's response to the publication of a memorandum of guidance (HSC(IS)32), by the Department of Health and Social Security, concerning the provision of family planning in the NHS. IN 1981, she wrote to her local Area Health Authority (AHA):

> 'Concerning the new DHSS *Guidelines* on the contraceptive and abortion treatment of children under both the legal and medical age of consent ... can I please ask you for a written assurance that in no circumstances whatsoever will any of my daughters ... be given contraceptive or abortion treatment whilst they are under sixteen ... without my knowledge, and irrefutable evidence of my consent (Emphasis added)
>
> (Kennedy & Grubb 1989: 3–4.)

The reply she received from the chairman of the AHA chose to frame the DoH circular to the same terms:

> 'We would expect our doctors to work within these *guidelines* but, as the Minister has stated, the final decision in these matters must be one of clinical judgement.' (Emphasis added).
>
> (Kennedy & Grubb 1989: 3–4.)

In taking her case to the Court of Appeal and finally to the House of Lords, Mrs Gillick contended that the advice contained in the 'guidelines' was morally flawed, and unlawful (*Gillick* 1985).

A recent statement from the Driver and Vehicle Licensing Agency entitled 'Fitness to drive: updated guidelines for cardiovascular fitness in vocational drivers' (Irvine & Petch 1994), revises the previous position stated in 'Fitness to drive: updated guidance on cardiac conditions in vocational and other professional drivers' (Gold & Oliver 1989). Although the current recommendations differ significantly from those they have replaced, it is not clear whether the authors' decision to replace 'guidance' with 'guidelines' in the later document confers any greater authority.

As we have seen in Chapters 2 and 5, the IoM wishes to restrict the term 'guideline' to systematically developed advisory statements created according to validated methodologies (Cluzeau *et al.* 1994). In the IoM's view, only those statements of clinical guidance that rest firmly upon the authority of science should be accorded the status of 'guidelines'. While this remains an important programmatic stance, clinicians, purchasers, patients and their lawyers require to know how to respond to the large number of heterogeneous guidelines already in circulation (Hurwitz 1995).

Clinical guidelines need to be understood generically as attempts to provide guidance on specific circumstances to practising doctors, in order to direct medical practice in one direction rather than another. As with a plumbline, a guideline can be heeded or not at the discretion of the clinician. However, a plumbline may only safely be ignored by a builder so long as the safety of a structure does not depend upon adherence to its guidance. When can a standard or guideline be safely ignored by a clinician? How do doctors recognise when a guideline constitutes an instruction to be carefully followed, cautiously ignored or safely disregarded? Can doctors be relied upon correctly to identify and reject bizarre and invalid standards, or guidelines emanating from sources which seek to impose factional interests upon medical practice (British Diabetic Association 1990)?

Guideline authority

In general terms, the authority of a guideline statement can be analysed in terms of its title to be believed, the standing of its developers and sponsors, and its moral grounding.

Title to be believed

A guideline's title to be believed reflects the credibility it is accorded by a relevant professional user group; clinicians, in the case of clinical guidelines. This credibility arises from an assessment of a variety of factors in the creation of the guideline including the following:

(1) The standard which the guideline purports to embody (for example, minimum or excellent practice).
(2) The sources acknowledged in the guideline's creation, the manner and systematic nature of the literature searches performed in its preparation.
(3) The quality of the available research and the strength of the evidence which the literature search may have marshalled in the guideline's preparation.
(4) The methodology adopted in the guideline's development, whether formal or informal, consensus based, or developed by systematic validated processes.
(5) The results of scientific evaluations of a guideline's effectiveness.

In varying degrees, such factors have a bearing upon a guideline's title to be believed, and hence upon the authority which it carries.

The guideline's sponsorship

A guideline gains a different type of authority from the professional standing of its development and sponsoring groups (which are not usually identical). Such authority derives from the respect in which the expertise, working practices and values of the guideline authors are held which, in turn, have an influence upon the standing of its authors in the eyes of relevant guideline user groups.

The capacity of a guideline's sponsoring organisation to influence others (perhaps by persuasion, perhaps by enforcement) confers additional authority. If the sponsoring body wields power, then whatever the intrinsic merit of a guideline (that is, whatever its title to be believed), the guideline is likely to take on some of the authority and power of the organisation which promulgates it. Asthma guidelines issued by the British Thoracic Society and diabetes care guidelines issued by the British Diabetic Association each individually carry the authority of their titles to be believed, but gain additional authority from the esteem in which their parent bodies are held (British Diabetic Association 1990; British Thoracic Society 1993).

The Department of Health's decision to adopt some guidelines in a drive to improve clinical effectiveness credits the guidelines with an official stamp of approval, adding an authority which stems from the NHS Management Executive's 'right to command' action in the NHS, and to enforce wide dissemination and even (though more contentiously) implementation (NHSME 1993).

Clinicians tend to focus upon a guideline's title to be believed in the belief that this is the major factor influencing implementation into practice. However, dissemination and implementation strategies also play a role (Eccles & Grimshaw 1995), as can sponsorship. Guidelines of poor title may be sponsored and distributed by third parties whose power to influence can be considerable, power that may inevitably affect how the guidelines are viewed. A guideline's influence may derive from a higher source than that of its sponsor, as with guidelines approved by the GMC. Currently awaiting greater delegated power from Parliament to investigate doctors' professional performance (Kilpatrick 1992), the GMC has shown an interest in 'approved guidelines' as embodying minimum standards of clinical care (GMC 1993).

Different sorts of guideline authority may enhance each other, as when effective guidelines of good title rebound positively on the reputation and influence of a sponsoring organisation. On the other hand, tensions may arise *between* different elements of authority, as when a prestigious organisation sponsors guidelines of variable quality and title (NHSME 1993).

Moral authority of guidelines

Because clinical guidelines currently comprise such a heterogeneous group of advisory statements, there can be no general moral duty for doctors to adhere to them. As we have seen, a guideline's authority is bound up with how clinicians evaluate and respond to the guidance it contains. Its authority is manifest by professional behaviour towards, and compliance with, its recommendations. For a responsible profession, therefore, authoritative guidelines, in order to *be* authoritative, must carry with them a transparent moral justification for implementation and use.

What sorts of moral justifications can be found to support the increasing calls for doctors to adhere to clinical guidelines? One attraction of the IoM's call to restrict what counts as a clinical guideline to only those recommendations grounded in formal scientific assessments of high quality research, is the increased transparency this gives to their moral authority. Because guidelines of this sort are likely to be valid, that is, to lead to the health gain predicted from their recommendations, it may be argued that doctors have the same moral duty to adhere to effective guidelines, as they do to employ efficacious medicines (Eddy 1990a). If either are likely to maximise patient benefit (cost effectively), an ethical imperative asserts itself which underpins much of clinical medicine (Gillon 1985).

But to which moral justification can we turn for the vast bulk of current guidelines, grounded as they are, in 'opinion or the musings of "expert" committees' (McDonald & Overhage 1994) rather than in controlled studies? Many standards and guidelines appear to be descriptive compilations of current practices. Following 'best practice', defined by consensus (assuming this consensus to be authentic) (Smith 1991) can provide patients with the security of knowing that their clinical care remains part of a collective enterprise. Healthcare informed by consensus guidelines helps to ensure that doctors meet their duty to provide treatment within an acceptable range of variation. Such a duty arises out of patients' reliance upon the medical profession (particularly in the context of a national health service) not offering atypical or idiosyncratic treatment which merely reflects the differing subjectivities of particular doctors or groups of doctors.

Recognition of unacceptable (and inexplicable) variability in the delivery of health services and resources has been one of the moral underpinnings of calls to establish standards, guidelines and protocols across wide areas of clinical activity (Hutchinson 1995). However, the 'guideline industry' now risks becoming a victim of the very problem it has been called upon to solve, namely unacceptable variability in validity. Consensus-based clinical guidelines recommend particular approaches to clinical problems with the moral authority of the law of averages. To some extent, they reflect a belief that:

> '... the true practice of medicine is learned from those with more experience. With a quick "let me show you the way this is done" a wealth of practical information is conveyed rapidly and effectively'
> (Swerdlow 1992.)

If the practice of medicine is correctly understood to be a life-long apprenticeship, it might be argued that, in certain circumstances, doctors have a duty to follow the practices of their teachers. In the absence of controlled studies this may be the safest moral approach; offering different medical care can amount to indulging in untested innovation. The problem, as Swerdlow (1992) has stated, is that:

> '... along with all this useful information comes a considerable burden of incorrect information with the status of lore ... Our charge is to determine what is best for our patients. We must, therefore, constantly question whether established medical practices have true benefit or if they are relics of the past or misconceptions of the present'.

Consensus-based guidelines could protect patients from clinical practices learned unthinkingly by apprenticeship from their teachers. However, the moral grounding here rests on the shaky assumption that a particular treatment approach is likely to be appropriate because this is the way a majority of doctors practise, or because 'opinion leaders', or clinicians of authority and standing practise in this way. But consensus can encompass a wide range of possible agreements from active assent or agreement under protest, to passive agreement and acquiescence. One American philosopher has argued that:

> '... medical practitioners should regard the recommendations of National Institutes of Health consensus development conferences as useful reference tools: not the rulings of philosopher-kings...'.
>
> (Tong 1991.)

A further danger in the creation and implementation of consensus guidelines lies in the possibility that their widespread use will fossilise customary practices. By encouraging a process of unthinking conformity, guideline-driven practice may lead to the destruction of change and innovation in medicine, and undermine clinical freedom. Doctors therefore need to guard against insistent demands for professional deference in the face of standards and guidelines from a new *dirigisme*:

> '... a view now ascendant among policymakers is that clinically based judgements that draw on a variety of formal and informal sources, as physicians' judgements traditionally have, are not as reliable a source of knowledge as those based on aggregated data. Thus a physician's individual, clinical experience is discounted, and aggregated data on behaviour and outcomes becomes the appropriate basis for choices in health care... The new faith in medical practice guidelines, managed care, and outcomes and health services research assumes that we can manipulate and generalize from such data: we know medicine sufficiently by knowing this information. Such a view enables, if not encourages, the progressive removal of medicine decisions from the bedside and from trained clinicians. This is a political story with enormous ramifications'.
>
> (Belkin 1994.)

The 'political story' to which the author here refers, is manifest as a tension between those standards and guidelines which emanate from self-regulation and the exercise of professional judgement, and guidelines and standards originating from external sources seeking to quell clinical freedom. Consensus guidelines and standards should not be allowed to drive out valid differences of approach to clinical care of patients.

Viewed as the medical profession's 'freedom to think ... freedom for initiative and individual responsibility' (Downie & Charlton 1992), clinical freedom has never been unfettered (Eddy 1990b; CSAG 1993). However, recognition and acceptance of clinical guidelines may amount to the medical profession welcoming a Trojan Horse into the privacy of the consultation. A GP who specialised in treating drug misusers without a framework adopted by Department of Health guidelines has stated that:

> 'In medicine, guidelines drawn up by the establishment are all too easily converted into regulations and a means of punishing dissenters'

> (Dally 1990.)

In *Dally v the GMC*, Dr Dally stood accused of serious professional misconduct in her prescribing of methadone and in failing to follow 'guidelines laid down for good clinical practice'. Although found not guilty of misconduct on account of breaching guidelines, her case anticipated that of an Australian GP in *Cranley v Medical Board of Western Australia* (*Cranley* 1992). In Dr Dally's view, the hearing was brought against her because she had dissented from a prevailing 'establishment' view of how drug addicts should be treated. Her treatment of opiate addicts had not accorded with the policy recommended by dangerous drug units in 1986, nor with the then Department of Health guidelines. The legal scholar and historian of the GMC, Russell Smith, agrees with her assessment, arguing that in *Dally v the GMC*:

> 'one was left with the unhappy situation of a doctor having her conduct adjudicated and its undesirability declared, presumably for the benefit of the whole medical community in knowing what was acceptable conduct in the eyes of the GMC, when she had merely been following one school of thought which had its own substantial body of advocates'

> (Smith 1994.)

There is clearly a danger that guidelines and standards issued by 'the authorities', whether represented by the Department of Health, the Royal Colleges or other organisations, will appear to possess a moral justification simply by virtue of the ensuing expectation that such guidelines will be complied with. It is important, therefore, to remember that standards can be contested, and compliance with guidelines, as in the case of *Early* (discussed in the introduction), may be challenged in law.

Legal authority of standards and guidelines

By enacting statutes which set in motion a framework to regulate clinical activities, legislative bodies can directly influence clinical standards.

United Kingdom statute
Statute aimed at regulating clinical activity may operate through the creation and empowerment of an organisation, as occurs in the Human

Fertilisation and Embryology Act 1990, or by special licensing arrangements as set up by the 1967 Abortion Act (as amended).

The Human Fertilisation and Embryology Act created the Human Fertilisation and Embryology Authority (HFEA) directing it to develop a Code of Practice 'for the proper conduct of activities'. HFEA has taken it upon itself to consult widely before 'deciding what our guidelines should say' (HFEA 1991). The resultant Code is an elaborate and wide-ranging document, covering 11 major areas of clinical practice, both setting and regulating ethical and clinical parameters of the provision of *in vitro* fertilisation in the UK. In accordance with the Act, the Code, and any subsequent revisions to it, has to be approved by the Secretary of State, who must lay it before Parliament before it can come into effect.

Department of Health regulations governing payments to GPs provide another example of clinical regulation, in this case backed by a statutory instrument (NHS 1992). Regulations spell out an 'organised programme' of care for patients with asthma or diabetes (DoH 1993). The resulting rules can be viewed as organisational guidelines for the clinical care of diseases in general practice and reveal another mode of Parliamentary influence upon clinical practice.

United States statute

In the US, major legislation seeking to regulate clinical activities by means of guidelines dates from the Peer Review Improvement Act 1982 which established peer review organisations (PROs) to ensure the quality and cost effectiveness of federally funded healthcare. PROs were empowered by Congress to develop criteria and norms by which to review all Medicare in-patient treatment, and to screen payment claims for evidence of poor quality of care. Congress responded to criticism of these criteria – very few providers being disqualified from reimbursement – by establishing the Agency for Health Care Policy Research (AHCPR) to 'enhance the quality, appropriateness, and effectiveness of health care services...' (Omnibus Reconciliation Act 1989). A new statute established a unit within the AHCPR, the Forum for Quality and Effectiveness in Health Care, composed of physicians, nurses and patients' representatives, whose brief is to commission clinical guidelines covering prevention, diagnosis and clinical management of important medical conditions.

The Act spells out the scope of the guidelines which are required to outline specific standards of quality together with clinical performance measures. The Forum does not itself develop guidelines (which are not intended to be Federal creations), though it does commission their development, updating and evaluation from public and private organisations, including professional and specialist medical associations. AHCPR guidelines do not, therefore, carry the force of law, though they have been produced as a result of legislation (Havinghurst 1990).

Standards, guidelines and the law of negligence

Civil actions in negligence evolved to meet a desire for vengeance for wrongs suffered as a result of non-criminal actions. In providing officially sanctioned compensation, the common law offered victims an alternative to that of taking the law into their own hands. Common law recognises that patients have a right to expect a certain standard of medical care. Conversely, doctors have a duty, enforceable in law, to provide clinical care that meets this standard. Can clinical guidelines have an influence upon the nature of this standard?

Under UK law, the standard of medical treatment a doctor owes to a patient was established in the case of *Bolam* (1957) in the words of McNair J: 'the test is the standard of the ordinary skilled man exercising and professing to have that special skill'. Although the duty of care is imposed by law, its standard is determined by the courts after hearing expert evidence. Doctors are required to act in a manner judged reasonable and proper by a body of other responsible doctors. In the words of Lord Scarman (speaking extrajudicially), the standard of medical care required by law is effectively 'set by the medical profession and is a totally medical proposition erected into a working rule of law' (Lord Scarman 1987). In *Bolam* (1957) the judge said:

> 'A doctor will not be guilty of negligence if he has acted in accordance with a practice accepted as proper by a responsible body of medical men skilled in that particular art.'

Expert testimony helps the courts to ascertain what is accepted and proper practice in specific cases. Although questions of breach of a doctor's duty are decided primarily on the basis of such expert evidence, Lord Bridge in *Sidaway* (1985), when applying the *Bolam* test did not accept that this could lead to the

> 'necessity "to hand over to the medical profession the entire question of the scope of this duty ... including the question of whether there has been a breach of that duty". Of course, if there is a conflict of evidence whether a responsible body of medical opinion approves ... in a particular case, the judge will have to resolve that conflict'.

Expert medical evidence is not therefore determinative. To be credible in court, expert witnesses require to have first-hand experience of the appropriate healthcare practice (Hodgkinson 1990; James 1995). In the case of *Early*, discussed in the introduction, the fact that the plaintiff's main expert witness was a *retired* anaesthetist may have influenced the judge's decision not to accord this evidence much weight.

Written standards or guidelines may be introduced to a UK court by an expert witness as evidence of accepted and customary standards of care, but they cannot be introduced as a substitute for expert testimony. Always wary of evidence which is not subject to cross examination, the courts would be likely to view guidelines as hearsay only (Howard & Crane 1982). The mere fact that a protocol exists for the care of a particular condition does not of itself establish the truth of its propositions, nor that compliance with the guideline would be reasonable in the circumstances, nor that non-compliance could amount to negligence. As stated in *Hunter* (1955):

> 'In the realm of diagnosis and treatment there is ample scope for genuine difference of opinion and one man is not negligent merely because his conclusion differs from that of other professional men.'

The case of the football fan, Tony Bland, provides an instance in which a court found that written guidelines drawn up by a responsible body of opinion can protect clinicians from liability in the eyes of the law (*Airedale NHS Trust* 1993). These guidelines were safeguards to be observed before discontinuing life support to patients in persistent vegetative state (PVS), developed by the Medical Ethics Committee of the BMA after wide-ranging consultation (BMA 1992). In his judgement, Lord Goff stated that:

> 'study of this document left me in no doubt that, if a doctor treating a PVS patient acts in accordance with the medical practice now being evolved by the Medical Ethics Committee of the BMA, he will be acting with the benefit of guidance from a responsible and competent body of professional opinion, as required by the *Bolam* test.'
>
> (*Airedale NHS Trust* 1993.)

According to the judgement, the BMA guidelines pass the *Bolam* test in the particular clinical circumstances of Tony Bland because they amount to 'guidance from a responsible body of professional opinion'. Since this is the standard of care required by law, compliance with the guidelines is compliance with the law. It is important to notice that the judgement recognises that the relevant guidance was 'being evolved'; courts appreciate that standards change over time. They may not, therefore, adopt an identical standard of care in otherwise identical future cases.

Standards, guidelines and consensus

In attempting to define minimum standards of care, the courts are not always able to rely upon the existence of medical consensus. Summarising the case of *Loveday v Renton and Wellcome Foundation Ltd* the editor of *Medical Law Reports* explained that the court held that failure to observe contraindication guidelines when administering whooping cough vaccination:

> 'would not in itself constitute negligence because there was a respectable and responsible body of medical opinion that some contraindications should not be observed because the risk of disease outweighed any actual or possible risk from the vaccine.'
>
> (*Loveday* 1990.)

Mere deviation from a guideline would be unlikely to be accepted as evidence of negligence by a UK court, unless the deviation itself was of a type which no doctor acting with ordinary skill and care would make (*Hunter* 1955). This principle of common law was invoked in *Cranley* (1992), involving alleged misconduct by an Australian GP. In prescribing injectable diazepam to heroin addicts, Dr Cranley deviated from guidance contained in the Australian National Methadone Guidelines and, as a consequence, was found guilty of 'infamous and improper conduct'. However, after hearing of a minority Australian medical opinion supporting treatment of opiate addicts within a harm reduction framework, as pursued by Dr Cranley, the Supreme Court of Western Australia upheld his appeal (*Cranley* 1992).

Standards of medical practice and the law

UK law holds that doctors have a responsibility to be aware of guideline statements which, in their field of practice, embody the minimum standard of care required by law. But which of the many clinical guidelines in existence possess this particular status? This question was addressed, with regard to the proliferation of published medical materials, by Denning LJ in the case of *Crawford v Board of Governors of Charing Cross Hospital*:

> 'it would be quite wrong to suggest that the medical man is negligent because he does not at once put into operation the suggestion that some contributor or other might make in a medical journal ... The time may come in a particular case when a new recommendation may be so well proved and so well known, and so well accepted that it should be adopted, but that was not so in this case'.
>
> (*Crawford* 1991.)

The key elements of Denning's test are: proof, dissemination, acceptance and adoption, each in combination with the notion of wide professional approval over time. Atypical or bizarre guidelines, and 'consensus' guidelines which fail to achieve professional acceptance, would be expected to fail this test and, more importantly, would likely fall foul of *Bolam*. A similar fate may await guidelines designed to hasten the incorporation of research findings into routine clinical care. Such guidelines, despite their possible scientific validity, could not be held representative of customary care until a variable period after publication and distribution (Haines & Jones 1994).

Courts have occasionally found professionally accepted standards of practice deficient, particularly in the area of how much information patients should be offered before they can validly express an informed consent to a procedure (*Clarke* 1989). In Australia, guidelines covering the provision of information to patients have been developed, and there have been calls for legislation to ensure such guidelines are admissible in court actions (Chalmers & Schwartz 1993).

In the USA, the state legislature in Maine has initiated a five-year experimental project to establish legally validated clinical guidelines admissible in court. The aim is to cut the cost of malpractice premiums and to retain doctors in high risk disciplines within the state (Edwards 1991). The process adopted has been set in motion by statute (Maine Public Law 1990) and designed by the Maine Medical Association, with the approval of the AHCPR and four national medical and surgical associations. Once guidelines and protocols have been developed and adopted by the Maine Licensing and Registration Boards, a doctor may cite the fact of having followed the guideline as an affirmative defence to a malpractice claim. Under this legislation, the standard of care embodied by the guideline temporarily becomes, through a process of judicial notice in court, the legally required standard of care. Because the legislation only allows Maine guidelines to be cited in a doctor's defence, deviation from such a guideline cannot yet be used by a plaintiff as presumptive evidence of negligence (Smith 1993). Arguably, asymmetry between the exculpatory (exonerating) value of guidelines to a doctor, and their lack of inculpatory (implicating) value to a patient, violates the need for 'due process and equal protection' (Mehlman 1990).

In one of the few surveys of actual guideline use in American medical malpractice actions, the authors report that in only 6.6% of actions do clinical guidelines play 'a relevant or pivotal role in the proof of negligence' (Hyams *et al.* 1995), but in two thirds of cases the guidelines were used for inculpatory purposes. The authors comment that: 'Education about the two-way use of practice guidelines in litigation should be a priority.'

Because the Maine legislation seems to confer immunity upon doctors who conform with certain guideline standards yet fails to increase the exposure of doctors choosing to ignore these guidelines, this law is open to the charge of being unconstitutional.

Discretion in relation to standards and guidelines

Rigid adherence to guidelines can be inappropriate, and lead to the erosion of clinical judgement and reduction of clinical practice to little more than a series of mechanistic rule-following procedures. The case of *McFarlane v Secretary of State for Scotland*, though itself concerned with correct administrative procedures rather than clinical decisions *per se*, nevertheless shows how a court can reverse too mechanistic an application of a guideline. Mr McFarlane appealed to the Sheriff Court in Scotland against a decision by the Secretary of State to revoke his driving licence after uncontested findings that his field of vision did not amount to the minimum recommended by the Royal College of Ophthalmologists, at least 20 degrees above and below the horizontal. The sheriff noted that the Secretary of State's adviser had 'simply followed the recommendations in the guidelines laid down' (*McFarlane* 1988). Further expert testimony centred on the congenital nature of the appellant's defect, which was neither degenerative nor progressive and to which he had fully adapted. McFarlane suffered from a left upper homonymous quadrantanopia, which it was deemed would have little significance to a driver looking straight ahead or from side to side in the rear mirror. He was not thought to be a danger to the public and his driving licence was duly reinstated.

The case highlights that advisory statements entitled 'guidance', 'guidelines' or 'recommendations' require to be interpreted by a proper exercise of discretion which, except in rare cases, should not be thought of as hard and fast rules.

> 'The law ... is prepared to allow decision-makers to develop and apply flexible guidelines to structure the exercise of their discretionary powers, provided they are not used rigidly so as to exclude the essence of discretion, namely a readiness to deal with each case on its merits.'
>
> (Cane 1992.)

The World Health Organization–International Society of Hypertension guidelines are explicit on the need for intelligent discretion in their use:

> 'Guidelines should not be seen as rigid constraints on a practising doctor's decisions. Guidelines should provide extensive, critical, and well balanced information on benefits and limitations of the various diagnostic and therapeutic interventions so that the physician may exert the most careful judgement in individual cases.'
>
> (WHO/ISH Mild Hypertension Liaison Committee 1993.)

Courts in the United States appreciate that guideline statements are frequently couched in terms which provide for considerable discretion on the part of clinicians. Deviation from clinical guidelines issued by an organisation as prestigious as the American Heart Association was found by a court to be acceptable as a result of unrefuted evidence that: 'American Heart Association's guidelines are mere guidelines that may be altered by the physician' (*Lowry* 1990).

Liability of guideline developers

Is it possible for guideline developers to be held liable if a patient suffers injury as a result of carelessly prepared guidelines? This issue did not arise directly in the case of *Early* and has not yet arisen as a substantive question in a UK court. However, third party liability for guideline statements has emerged in several contexts in the United States. In *Wickline v California* a court held that:

> 'third party payers ... can be held legally accountable when medically inappropriate decisions result from defects in the design or implementation of cost containment mechanisms.'
>
> (*Wickline* 1986.)

The case involved early discharge of a patient according to a Medi-Cal utilisation review protocol consisting of treatment guidelines, including length of stay criteria, approved for payment purposes. It was alleged that as a result of early discharge, the patient later had to undergo an amputation.

In *Wickline*, the patient's doctor had complied with the particular guideline without protest. The court decided that a doctor could not claim as a defence to negligence, that his or her clinical judgement had been corrupted by clinical guidelines.

> '[A] physician who complies without protest ... when his medical judgement dictates otherwise, cannot avoid responsibility for his patient's care.'
>
> (*Wickline* 1986.)

However, in *Wilson v Blue Cross of California* an appeal court held that a doctor's failure to protest against inappropriate review rules in the case of a patient harmed by adherence to these rules did *not* automatically protect the review organisation from liability. The case involved a depressed patient who committed suicide after early discharge from hospital as a result of a decision by Blue Cross to refuse payment for any further hospital care. The court found that:

> 'a decision not to approve further hospitalization was a substantial factor in bringing about the decedent's demise.'
>
> (*Wilson* 1990.)

In the USA, therefore, it seems likely that developers and issuers of clinical guidelines could be held liable if adherence to substandard guidelines are found to be a proximate cause of harm suffered by a patient.

Conclusion

In his Shattuck Lecture to the Massachusetts Medical Society in 1988, Paul Ellwood said:

> 'A system of appropriate medical standards, guidelines, and hard-and-fast rules that can be used by physicians in caring for their patients – referred to by many physicians as "cookbook medicine" – continues to be devastatingly controversial, providing a bonanza for litigators, a conundrum when patients do not fit the standards, a bureaucrat's paradise, and the last stand for free physicians.'
>
> (Ellwood 1988.)

This chapter has shown that any authority which a clinical guideline may possess results from a complex mosaic of assessments: from valuations of its title to be believed, to its moral authority, the results (if any) of effectiveness studies, and the authority it may gain by virtue of sponsorship. The legal status of a guideline depends on whether its creation has statutory backing and whether it accurately represents practice which is accepted by a responsible body of doctors.

Ellwood's claim that standards and guidelines will provide 'a bonanza for litigators' has so far proved wide of the mark. In actions for medical negligence, the required standard of medical care is neither the best nor necessarily the most effective medical practice. In the UK, the standard is defined and evaluated on the basis of an assessment by a judge (jury in the USA) of evidence which emerges from the testimony of medical experts. Experts elucidate the standard of the medical profession in the relevant area of practice.

Guideline statements offer the courts explicit and compressed examples of standards for a wide array of complex clinical activities. Their continued proliferation means that guidelines will increasingly feature in actions alleging medical negligence, but admission of protocols and guidelines as evidence of clinical standards has not short-circuited the common law principles by which the courts come to a view. The courts have not slavishly followed standards enunciated in guidelines without critically evaluating their authority, applicability and flexibility according to accepted common law principles.

Guidelines are also conspicuous features of the changed regulatory structure of healthcare. Lomas (1993) believes that:

> 'practice guidelines are, in fact, policies insofar as a policy is a rule to establish, control, or change the behaviour of institutions, individuals, or both'.

In Lomas's view, the development of most clinical guidelines must be judged, on the basis of policy-making standards, as 'decidedly primitive' and under-developed. The processes of clinical guideline development and implementation have much to learn from equivalent processes in the domain of public policy legislation.

Clinical policy making has almost always been accomplished informally, by largely unwritten processes unavailable to public view and debate. By contrast, public policy legislation procedures are usually written down, with policy being developed by formal processes of consultation and public debate. In the view of Lomas (1993), because legislation in western democracies necessarily involves

> 'accountability and responsivity to available estimates of the facts (evidence), interested parties' interpretations of the facts (vested interests), and the relative priority afforded to the facts (values)'

it provides a powerful model for the formation and implementation of clinical guidelines.

If clinical standards and guidelines are to be accorded a profound and pervasive regulatory role in the delivery of healthcare, their development and implementation require to be made accountable. For explicit standards and guidelines to be safely adopted, rejected or appropriately ignored, their medical, moral and legal authority must be scrutinised and understood.

References

Airedale NHS Trust (1993) *Airedale NHS Trust v Bland (Guardian ad litem)*, 1 All ER 821.

Anonymous (1991a) Guidelines for writing papers. *British Medical Journal* **302**: 40.

Anonymous (1991b) Guidelines for referees. *British Medical Journal* **302**: 41.

Belkin, G.S. (1994) Numbers and the politics of health care. *Journal of Health Politics, Policy and Law* **19**: 3–5.

BMA (1992) *Discussion Paper on Treatment of Patients in Persistent Vegetative State*, Medical Ethics Committee, British Medical Association, London.

Bolam (1957) *Bolam v Friern Hospital Management Committee*, 2 All ER 118–28 at 122.

British Diabetic Association (1990) *Guidelines for the Development and Integration of General Practitioner Care of Diabetes with Hospital Based Systems*, British Diabetic Association, London.

British Thoracic Society (1993) Guidelines on the Management of Asthma. Statement by the British Thoracic Society, the British Paediatric Association, the Research Unit of the Royal College of Physicians of London, the King's Fund Centre, the National Asthma Campaign, the Royal College of General Practitioners, the General Practitioners in Asthma Group, the British Association of Accident and Emergency Medicine, and the British Paediatric Respiratory Group following a meeting at the Royal College of Physicians, London on 4–5 June 1992. *Thorax* **48** (Suppl.): S1–S24.

Cane, P. (1992) *An Introduction to Administrative Law*, Clarendon Press, Oxford.

Chalmers, A. (1994) *Samuel Johnson's Dictionary of the English Language*, Studio Editions Ltd, London.

Chalmers, D. & Schwartz, R. (1993) *Rogers v Whitaker* and informed consent in Australia: a fair dinkum duty of disclosure, *Medical Law Review* **1**: 139–59.

Chalmers, I. (1994) Why are opinions about health care so often wrong? *Medico-legal Journal* **62**: 116–30.

Clarke (1989) *Clarke v Adams (1950)*, quoted in: Kennedy, I. & Grubb, A., *Medical Law, Text and Materials*, Butterworths, London.

Cluzeau, F., Littlejohns, P. & Grimshaw, J. (1994) Appraising clinical guidelines: towards a *Which?* guide for purchasers. *Quality in Health Care* **3**: 121–2.

Cranley (1992) *Cranley v Medical Board of Western Australia* (Sup Ct WA), 3 Med LR 94–113.

Crawford (1991) *Crawford v Board of Governors of Charing Cross Hospital (1953)*, In: *Law and Medical Ethics* (eds J. Mason & R. McCall Smith), Butterworths, London.

CSAG (1993) *Access to and Availability of Specialist Services*, Clinical Standards Advisory Group, HMSO, London.

CSAGC (1994) *Standards of Clinical Care for People with Diabetes*. Report of the Clinical Standards Advisory Group Committee and the Government response. HMSO, London.

Dally, A. (1990) *A Doctor's Story*, Macmillan, London.

DoH (1993) *The National Health Service Statement of Fees and Allowances*, Paragraph 30, Schedules 4 and 5, Department of Health and Welsh Office 1993, London.

Downie, R.S. & Charlton, B.G. (1992) *The Making of a Doctor*, Oxford University Press, Oxford.

Early (1994) *Early v Newham Health Authority*. *Medical Law Review* **5**: 215–17.

Eccles, M. & Grimshaw, J. (1995) The implementation of guidelines in general practice. In: *The Development and Implementation of Clinical Guidelines. Report From General Practice* (ed. R. Baker). Royal College of General Practitioners, London, pp. 12–15.

Eddy, D.M. (1990a) Practice policies: where do they come from? *Journal of the American Medical Association* **263**: 1265–75.

Eddy, D.M. (1990b) Designing a practice policy, standards, guidelines and options. *Journal of the American Medical Association* **263**: 3077–84.

Edwards, D. (1991) The Maine 5-year medical demonstration project. Presentation at the agency for health care policy and research confidence on medical liability issues, Washington, DC. In: *Guidelines for Clinical Practice* (eds. M. Field & K. Low), National Academy Press, Washington, DC, 1992, p. 130.

Ellman, R. (1989) Motor mania: physician regulation runs amok. *Loyola University Chicago Law Journal* **20**: 721–73.

Ellwood, P.M. (1988) Shattuck Lecture – outcomes management, a technology of patient experience. *New England Journal of Medicine* **318**: 1549–56.

Feder, G. (1994) Clinical guidelines in 1994. *British Medical Journal* **309**: 1457–8.

Field, M. & Lohr, K. (eds) (1990) *Clinical Practice Guidelines: Directions for a New Program*, Institute of Medicine, National Academy Press, Washington, DC.

Gillick (1985) *Gillick v West Norfolk and Wisbech Area Health Authority*, 3 All ER 402.

Gillon, R. (1985) *Philosophical Medical Ethics*, John Wiley & Sons, Chichester.

GMC (1993) The use of drugs to assist weight loss. *GMC News Review* **3**: 2.

Gold, R. & Oliver, M. (1989) Fitness to drive: updated guidance on cardiac conditions in vocational drivers and other drivers. *Health Trends* **21**: 88–9.

Haines, A. & Jones, R. (1994) Implementing the findings of research. *British Medical Journal* **308**: 1488–92.

Havinghurst, C. (1990) Practice guidelines for medical care: the policy rationale. *St Louis University Law Journal* **34**: 777–819.

Healthcare Standards Directory (1993) Quoted in: Leone, A. Medical practice guidelines are useful tools in litigation. *Medical Malpractice: Law and Strategy* **10**: 1–6.

HFEA (1991) Letter accompanying the *Code of Practice*, Human Fertilisation and Embryology Authority, Document ref CH (91), London.

Hodgkinson, T. (1990) *Expert Evidence: Law and Practice*, Sweet & Maxwell, London.

Holmes, O.W. (1903), quoted in: Medical standard setting in the current malpractice environment, *University of California at Davis Law Review* (1989) **22**: 423.

Hopkins, A. (1993) Audit and accountability. In: *Eighty-five Not Out. Essays to Honour Sir George Godber* (ed. S. Lock), King Edward's Hospital Fund for London, London.

Howard, M. & Crane, P. (1982) *Phipson on Evidence*, Sweet & Maxwell, London.

Hunter (1955) *Hunter v Hanley 1955 SC 200 (Court of Session)*, Quoted in: Kennedy, I. & Grubb, A. (1989) *Medical Law, Text and Materials*, Butterworths, London, 420.

Hurwitz, B. (1995) Guidelines effectiveness – the pitfalls and obstacles. In: *The Development and Implementation of Clinical Guidelines. Report from General Practice* (ed. R. Baker) Royal College of General Practitioners, London.

Hutchinson, A. (1995) Improving the quality of health care – the place of clinical guidelines. In: *The Development and Implementation of Clinical Guidelines* (ed. R. Baker), Royal College of General Practitioners, London, pp. 1–2.

Hyams, A.L., Brandenurg, J.A., Lipsitz, S.R., Shapiro, D.W. & Brennan, T.A. (1995) Practice guidelines and malpractice litigation: a two-way street. *Annals of Internal Medicine* **122**: 450–55.

Irvine, J. & Petch, M. (1994) Fitness to drive: updated guidelines for cardio-vascular fitness in vocational drivers. *Health Trends* **26**: 38–40.

James, D.L. (1995) Limitations of expert evidence. Conference report. *Journal of the Royal College of Physicians of London* **1**: 50–52.

Kennedy, I. (1993) Medicine in society, now and in the future. In: *Eighty-five Not Out. Essays to Honour Sir George Godber* (ed. S. Lock), King Edward's Hospital Fund for London, London.

Kennedy, I. & Grubb, L. (1989) *Medical Law, Text and Materials*, Butterworth & Co., London.

Kilpatrick, R. (1992) President's Foreword. In: *Annual Report of the General Medical Council*, General Medical Council, London, pp. 1–4.

Leone, A. (1993) Medical practice guidelines are useful tools in litigation. *Medical Malpractice: Law and Strategy* **10**: 1–6.

Lomas, J. (1993) Making clinical policy explicit. *International Journal of Technology Assessment in Health Care* **9**: 11–25.

Lord Scarman (1987) Law and medical practice. In: *Medicine in Contemporary Society* (ed. P. Byrne). King Edward's Hospital Fund for London, London.

Loveday (1990) *Loveday v Renton and Wellcome Foundation Ltd (QBD)*, 1 Med LR 117–204.

Lowry (1990) *Lowry v Henry Mayo Newall Memorial Hospital (CA)*, 229– Cal Rptr 620.

Maine Public Law (1990) No. 1990 Ch 931, 24 MRSA 2972–2978. Cited in: Mehlman, M.J., Assuring the quality of medical care: the impact of outcome measurement and practice standards. *Law Medical Health Care* **18**: 384, reference 113.

McDonald, C.J. & Ovehage, J.M. (1994) Guidelines you can follow and can trust. *Journal of the American Medical Association* **271**: 872–3.

McFarlane (1988) *McFarlane v Secretary of State for Scotland*, Scottish Civil Law Reports 623–8.

McKee, M. & Clarke, A. (1995) Guidelines, enthusiasms, uncertainty and the limits to purchasing. *British Medical Journal* **310**: 101–104.

Mehlman, M.J. (1990) Assuring the quality of medical care: the impact of outcome measurement and practice standards. *Law Med Health Care* **18**: 378.

National Health and Medical Research Council Working Party (1991). General guidelines for medical practitioners on providing information to patients. Australian government publication service 1991, referenced in Chalmers, D. & Schwartz (1993) *Rogers v Whitaker* and informed consent in Australia: a fair dinkum duty of disclosure *Medical Law Review* **1**: 139–59.

NHS (1992) *The National Health Service (General Medical Services) Regulations 1992*, HMSO, London.

NHSME (1993) *Improving Clinical Effectiveness*, EL(93)115, Annex B, NHS Management Executive, Department of Health, Leeds.

Omnibus Reconciliation Act (1989) Public Law 101–239. In *Clinical Practice Guidelines: Directions for a New Program* (eds M. Field & K. Lohr). Institute of Medicine, National Academy Press, Washington, DC, 1990, pp. 107–27.

Sidaway (1985) *Sidaway v Board of Governors of the Bethlem and the Maudsley Hospital*, 1 All ER 643.

Silver, G. (1987) Discordant priorities. *Lancet* i: 1195.

Smith, G.H. (1993) A case study in progress: practice guidelines and the affirmative defense in Maine. *Journal of Quality Improvement* **19**, 355–62.

Smith, R. (1991) Where is the wisdom...? The poverty of medical evidence. *British Medical Journal* **303**: 798–9.

Smith, R.G. (1994) *Medical Discipline, the Professional Conduct Jurisdiction of the General Medical Council 1858–1990*, Oxford Clarendon Press, Oxford.

Swerdlow, P.S. (1992) A tradition of testing ironclad practices. *Journal of the American Medical Association* **267**: 560–61.

Tong, R. (1991) The epistemology and ethics of consensus: uses and misuses of 'ethical' expertise. *Journal of Medicine and Philosophy* **16**: 409–26.

WHO/ISH Mild Hypertension Liaison Committee (1993) Summary of 1993 World Health Organization–International Society of Hypertension guidelines for the management of mild hypertension. *British Medical Journal* **307**: 1541–6.

Wickline (1986) *Wickline v California*, 228 Cal Rptr 661, 667.

Wilson (1990) *Wilson v Blue Cross of California*, 222 Cal App 3d 660.

10 ◆ Partnerships in Clinical Audit: Senior NHS Management and the Clinical Professions

David Bowden

Introduction

As we move increasingly from a tradition of clinical freedom to evidence-based medicine, relationships will change; relationships between clinicians and patients, between the differing clinical professions and, vitally, between clinicians and managers.

The past ten years have seen quite dramatic changes, for managers and clinicians alike. For both, the pressures have increased, in different ways, but to the same end – to achieve more and improved patient care. This in turn has led to pressure and tension in relationships between clinicians and managers. In many cases, this has been creative and has resulted in a more dynamic and innovative environment. In other situations, it has been less constructive.

It is vital that clinicians and managers recognise more explicitly the pressures under which each other is placed. Each needs to be more honest and open with the other and each needs to share anxieties and talk through options for change with the other. They need to be clear about the balance between clinical autonomy and managerial control, to agree on the priorities for action and resources, accept the value of each other's contribution, work together to identify and manage the systems failures which lead to patient damage, and be more proactive and positive in the identification and implementation of each other's decisions. Each needs to ensure that, while they have different imperatives, both work to a common agenda.

To achieve this, managers must develop and create a supportive, encouraging, blame-free culture, where professionals and other staff feel valued for their contribution. In response, clinicians must accept that managers must, and will, monitor the clinical effectiveness of treatments and care. Managers must also satisfy themselves that the professions have adequate mechanisms to police themselves and to make changes to rectify inadequacies and unsafe practice, and will need to assure themselves about individual levels of competence and performance.

Clinical audit

The need for a partnership between clinicians and managers in guaranteeing the success of clinical audit is crucial, not least because it has an important part to play in the process of establishing the appropriateness, effectiveness and efficiency of clinical interventions, treatments, investigations and care as Chapters 1–4 have shown. Indeed, clinical audit is already proving to be of great importance to the fate of provider organisations in the NHS; they will thrive or fail because of the quality of the care they give, as well as because of the cost and accessibility of that care. Furthermore, success or failure will depend not only on the quality of the clinical service itself, but on a Trust's ability to *prove* to purchasers that its clinicians are providing an effective, quality service which meets patients' satisfaction.

There will continue to be impositions which require quality of care to be related to the quantity and cost of that care. More explicit clinical quality standards and outcome measures will be specified in contracts between health authorities and their providers. The process for developing quality standards is as follows:

(1) Step 1 – define service objectives:
   - health benefits
   - components of clinical workload
   - outcome orientated goals
   - service specification.
(2) Step 2 – define quality standards for each goal:
   - top down or bottom up?
   - imposed or peer review?
   - structure/process/outcome
   - measurable/realistic/acceptable.
(3) Monitor.

Doctors and managers will be required to share clinical audit information within agreed rules of confidentiality and managers will generally want to show the value of their being involved in the audit process.

Clinical audit should be seen as a natural progression of medical audit or, indeed, of any of the other single professional peer-review processes. The prime purpose of medical audit should always have been to enable the professionals concerned to analyse systematically and critically the quality of their individual treatments and that of their medical colleagues. Clinical audit has the benefit of being a more patient-focused process involving all members of the clinical care team in a multidisciplinary assessment and review of the overall effect of their collective clinical activities on the outcome of the care provided. As such, it should increasingly create opportunities to identify and analyse the suitability and safeness of the various processes of care and the clinical systems which support them. Some may require formalisation through care plans, clinical protocols or even clinical pathways, as Bentley *et al.* discuss in Chapter 7. What is so important is that the organisation creates real opportunities both to initiate such requirements, and to review their value. Clinical audit is: a study of various aspects of the structure, process and outcome of clinical care, carried out by those personally engaged in the activity concerned, in order to measure whether predetermined objectives and standards have been attained, so as to assess the quality of care delivered.

Clinical audit and risk management

Clinical audit is part of clinical risk management, as Miles *et al.* showed in Chapter 1. It is best described in this context as a process for the identification, evaluation and management of those risks which occur outside the clinical team, which have a significant adverse impact on the clinical team's activities, but over which the clinical team has no control. Audit, risk management and quality improvement require the following:

(1) Medical audit, a peer-review process enabling doctors to systematically and critically analyse the quality and outcome of their treatment.
(2) Clinical audit, a patient-focused audit process involving doctors, nurses and other clinicians who comprise the clinical care team.
(3) Risk management, a process for the identification of risks which have adverse effects on the quality of care and the safety of patients, staff and visitors; the assessment and evaluation of those risks; and the taking of positive action to eliminate or reduce them.
(4) Quality assurance, working throughout the organisation towards improving and maintaining the quality of care to patients. See Figure 10.1 for an illustrative version of this construct.

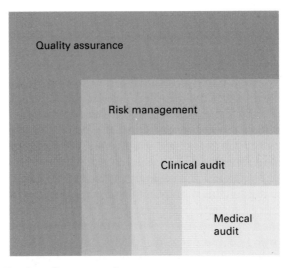

Fig. 10.1 Total quality approach.

By its very nature, healthcare is a risky activity. Indeed, doctors and other health professionals should not be discouraged from taking some risks in developing more effective methods of treatment. However, such risks should be taken as a result of a positive decision to do so, on the basis of good information and a sound understanding of the possible consequences and likely outcome of treatment. Wherever possible, this should be done with the knowledge and consent of the patient concerned.

What is of concern is the wide range of risks which occur by accident rather than design. Even more worrying are those untoward incidents which result from a lack of clear policies, deficient working practices, poorly defined responsibilities, inadequate communications and people working beyond their competence. The challenge for clinicians and health service managers alike is to eliminate, or at least reduce, the potential for such misfortunes by being more proactive in the future management of risk. Clinicians manage a great many risk situations every day, but on an *ad hoc* basis and in an unco-ordinated way. What needs to be recognised is that there are major benefits to be gained in doing so in a more co-ordinated, systematic and focused way.

So, risk management, as with clinical audit, has two dimensions – proactive and reactive. The reactive approach is based on a retrospective analysis of reported adverse incidents, mistakes and 'near misses', and on ensuring that the corrective actions are taken to prevent recurrence. In this approach, there are several warning signs which can lead to effective management of risk, and the following events should always be reported and logged on the adverse incident or clinical audit database:

- unexpected or trauma related death
- neurological deficit not present on admission
- coma not present on admission
- disfigurement present on discharge, not present on admission, including amputation
- unplanned return to the operating theatre
- unplanned admission to ICU
- failure to act on imaging or pathology result
- imaging or pathology report to wrong patient
- adverse medication problem
- equipment failure leading to patient injury
- swab/instrument count incorrect at end of operation
- absent medical notes.

This is an enormously beneficial mechanism for enhancing the safety of patient care. Clinical audit should also ensure that it contains a facility for retrospective review through

- learning of lessons
- correction of errors/implementation of change
- prevention of recurrence

- analysis of variances and adverse incidents
- future control and containment of variance.

The proactive approach is concerned with ensuring that the existing deficiencies in the care processes are clearly identified *before* they cause harm or an ineffective outcome; that the clinical team assesses positively the potential for future systems failure; that it analyses the priorities for action; and that it initiates action to eliminate or reduce the deficiencies in the future.

Involvement of senior managers in the audit process

In the past, managers have largely watched the development of clinical audit from the sidelines, partly because of clinicians' sensitivity about the issue and partly because of managers' preoccupation with a wealth of other changes that have occurred in the past few years. But as clinical audit becomes more important to how they manage their organisation, Trust managers can no longer afford to be content with the status of spectator. They will want to be involved players in a genuine partnership with clinical colleagues. In forming that partnership, it will be necessary to establish what managers can and should do to stimulate the clinical audit process. Similarly, they must be clear about what information managers will expect to receive from that process, and why. An indication of what is needed is given in Table 10.1.

What managers should do for audit

Environment

General managers have a responsibility to provide a suitable environment for audit and, where clinical audit does not exist, an obligation to take the lead by giving top level commitment to developing a formal process. Experience shows that an incremental, evolutionary, non-punitive and participative peer-review approach is more readily accepted than a system imposed by management.

The Trust board also has an important role. Not only must it endorse and support the clinical audit initiative, but it must also define its priorities in relation to the controversial quality versus quantity debate. The board needs to be explicit about whether it is prepared to condone a situation where the quality of patient care is being compromised, in comparison to its own predetermined standards. If so, with whom should it share that established position? If not, what implications might this have for cost and activity? There is a clear requirement for the board not only to ensure that such difficult issues are addressed in a focused way, but also that it creates a specific set of criteria which will guide future decision making on resource allocation and standard setting. Of equal importance is the need to inform clinicians how they should interpret these judgements, particularly with regard to the admission of emergency patients into overstretched services.

Table 10.1 Past and future characteristics of clinical audit

Characteristic	Past	Future
Participation of doctors	Entirely voluntary, so dominated by enthusiasts. Mainly concerned with medical audit.	Almost compulsory, through peer pressure, job plans, clinical directorates, pressure from other members of clinical team, and contracting process.
Participation of other healthcare processionals	Limited participation, except perhaps in data collection.	Widespread participation in planning systems and collecting and analysing data.
Participation of managers	Little management involvement or interest.	Audit central to management objectives; managers involved and interested.
Planning and development of audit systems	Unco-ordinated, led by individual clinicians, lacking comparability.	Co-ordinated by clinicians and managers. Integrated with general information strategies.
Relevance to organisation's objectives	Peripheral to objectives as defined by review processes, Trust policies, etc.	Central to organisation's objectives, as defined by contracting process. Important for organisation's viability/ success.
Effect on organisation's performance	Little effect on performance – few changes in individual or group clinical working practices.	Measurable and continuing effect on organisation's performance – clinically and managerially.

Cultural change

The boundaries which have sometimes existed between various clinical professions have often led to an unwillingness on the part of some practitioners to share fully their personal uncertainties, fallibilities and deficiencies with colleagues of other professions within the same clinical team (McIntyre 1995). That these have already been identified implicitly is often ignored or avoided by the practitioner concerned, and for clinical audit to thrive, this cannot be allowed to continue. Self audit requires a willingness by team members, of whatever level, to admit individual mistakes and inadequacies. It requires openness and honesty between all members of the clinical team and demands a positive approach to put things right. As a result, attitudes and behaviour may have to change and there is a necessity for the most senior managers in the Trust to encourage a supportive and non-punitive approach, rather than one of recrimination and blame. The most effective chief executives will be those who state explicitly what is the culture of the organisation in this respect, so that no one is in any doubt.

Resources

Audit cannot be undertaken sensibly and comprehensively without proper support and allocated resources. The regular review of consultant job plans provides an ideal opportunity for managers to acknowledge the importance of audit by allocating specific sessional time for doctors. Similar consideration should be given to all other clinical staff. This will make the quality–quantity trade off more explicit, maybe with the consequence that some clinics or theatre sessions are forfeited. Resources are also needed to pay for specific research activities and for study leave. Funds must be made available to purchase the necessary information systems and to provide technical and administrative support staff.

Clinical audit should not be seen as a cheap, peripheral activity, but rather as an integral component of good professional practice (see Chapter 1). It needs time, staff and money to develop a proper, comprehensive approach. Of course, such investments must be shown to result in improved outcomes and better patient care (Miles 1995a), as well as making the work of clinicians more professionally rewarding.

Information systems

Together, clinicians and managers should be developing and facilitating the introduction of new techniques in audit and information systems which are a key tool in audit (Wyatt 1994a–c; 1995). As the volume and complexity of clinical audit activity increases, the information needs of clinical audit will need to be integrated into corporate information strategies. While the sense of clinical ownership of the information must not be lost, clinical audit activities, risk management, clinical effectiveness, contracting and other management processes will benefit from the use of a shared database.

Incentives for audit

The contracting mechanism should provide incentives for providers to meet agreed workload targets at lower overall costs than the specified contract price, without adversely affecting the quality standards identified. This may be achieved by developing more efficient systems of working, such as those advanced by Bentley *et al.* in Chapter 7. When costs are reduced, it should be possible to retain the funds saved for use by the clinical departments concerned.

Similarly, there is a need to create systems of incentive to reward clinicians achieving improvements in clinical outcomes, with the emphasis on recognising improved performances rather than imposing sanctions to penalise under-achievers.

Peer-review audit and patient satisfaction

Managers are required, where necessary, to provide the interface between standard setting based on internal peer review (looking at patient care from within the organisation) and standards of patient satisfaction (looking at the organisation from the outside). In so doing, they may well need to be involved in helping to reconcile the potentially conflicting viewpoints of clinicians and patients on some issues, as Rigge explains in Chapter 11.

Confidentiality

With litigation for clinical negligence and malpractice increasing in frequency, managers have a responsibility to establish guidelines on confidentiality of clinical information within the organisation and outside it. The guidelines should have the twin aims of preserving clinical confidence and using audit information properly. They should also determine the rights of access of different staff groups to the audit information.

In summary, managers must give a lead, and ensure appropriate staffing, funding and support to make it easier and more rewarding for clinicians to perform their duties. They should not seek to interfere with the individual professional's clinical judgements, but rather ensure an increasing focus on evidence-based healthcare provision. This is best achieved by managers and clinicians working more closely as partners.

What managers expect and need from audit

Access to information

Managers in both commissioning authorities and provider Trusts need information to determine the quality of the clinical services being provided and to assess which clinical activities and treatments actually produce the most effective outcomes. That information should not only identify the standards related to the processes used in the departments concerned but, increasingly, must compare the predicted and actual outcomes of those activities. Information is also required to allow managers to assess how well the audit programmes are working and whether they are meeting the overall objective of producing better patient care. While most managers will be committed to supporting audit, they will be reluctant to see resources devoted to it if it does not produce measurable benefits for patients (Miles 1995a).

Audit in contracting between purchaser and provider

Without doubt, the health authorities, as commissioners of clinical services, are establishing progressively more advanced quality standards in the service contracts they agree with Trusts. Increasingly, GP fundholders will have similar aims in their contracting process. This will force the providers to demonstrate not only that they have formalised audit programmes in place but also that they meet the jointly agreed treatment standards.

There is also concern to develop the commissioning mechanism through an increasing focus on guideline-based purchasing, an approach recommended by some (Sheldon & Borowitz 1993), but incurring warnings from others (Miles 1995b; see also Chapter 8). Trusts which cannot match these expectations may well not be asked to provide the services in the future.

Audit and managing the organisation

The establishment of clinical directorates has created an increasingly powerful position for clinicians within Trusts. They are empowered with much control and authority for managing the resources used within their directorates, and collectively the clinical directors should be in a position to influence significantly and more directly the running of the whole organisation.

The clinical director is pivotal to the management of the service as he combines professional knowledge with managerial clout, but the directors need clinical audit information to support their decisions and actions. All too often, audit has been the missing third leg of the performance–management tripod which relates activity to costs and quality. The chief executive expects to see all three elements being managed together in directorates, with clinical audit and the management of resources converging to provide real evidence of value for money. The key to this is that the clinical director should be accountable for ensuring that there is a totally integrated management of quality, quantity, and cost; cost effectiveness and clinical effectiveness must be linked (Drummond 1995). Running a directorate more efficiently both releases and generates more resources which can be used to maximise clinical practices in determining the quality of service provided, as Chapter 7 points out.

It follows that clinical audit programmes must be based in the individual directorates and their effectiveness must be a key responsibility of the clinical director. Unless he believes in their value and owns the process, then the time, money and effort which is devoted to the programmes will gradually and inexorably diminish in their impact. It is no longer enough for clinicians or managers alike to satisfy themselves that clinical audit is being practised simply because there is a Trust clinical audit committee.

The place of audit within patient-focused care

With many Trusts creating different models of patient-focused care, the senior managers have an obligation to ensure that the clinical audit process is directly involved and used in that wide-ranging concept. Patient-focused care means:

- making services suit the patient(s), rather than the reverse
- focusing the care process on the individual patient
- making the process of planning and delivering care more clearly defined
- reducing the number of individual interventions in the delivery of care
- ensuring a co-ordinated and integrated approach to the care process
- ensuring improved integration and continuity of care
- minimising patient movement within the hospital/system
- providing safe, effective and efficient patient care.

An essential ingredient in this approach is the establishment of care pathways. These involve: a multidisciplinary process of patient-focused care which specifies key events, tests and assessments, occurring in a timely fashion to produce the best prescribed outcomes, within the resources and activities available, for an appropriate episode of care. Clinical audit has vital inputs to make both proactively in the development of the care pathway, and retrospectively in assessing the variances from the predicted activity (Figure 10.2). The chief executive will wish to create a monitoring system to establish the effectiveness of that process.

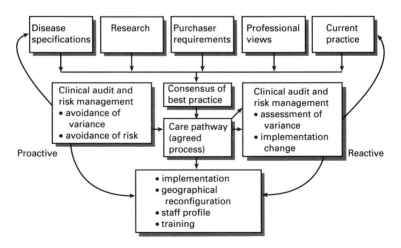

Fig. 10.2   Patient-focused care.

Conclusion

In conclusion, clinical audit is going to matter in future – to managers and clinicians in provider organisations, to commissioning groups and, most importantly, to patients. It will be crucial to the success and viability of Trusts in the NHS, and so managers and clinicians have to work together to develop effective programmes. Clinicians should seize the opportunity to be much more involved in shaping the quality of provider services, as key parts of a multi-professional team. Managers should rise to the challenge of becoming better educated and better informed about the work of their clinical colleagues and between them they really can make clinical audit start to count.

References

Bowden, D. (1995) Is clinical practice improved by risk management? *Journal of Evaluation in Clinical Practice* **1**: 77–9.

Drummond, M. (1995) The role of health economics in clinical evaluation. *Journal of Evaluation in Clinical Practice* **1**: 71–5.

McIntyre, N. (1995) Evaluation in clinical practice: problems, principles and precedents. *Journal of Evaluation in Clinical Practice* **1**: 5–13.

Miles, A. (1995a) Critical inquiry into clinical practice. *Journal of Evaluation in Clinical Practice* **1**: 3–4.

Miles, A. (1995b) Purchasing quality in clinical practice – what on earth do we mean? *Journal of Evaluation in Clinical Practice* **1**: 81–4.

Sheldon, T. & Borowitz, M. (1993) Changing the measure of quality in the NHS: from purchasing activity to purchasing protocols. *Quality in Health Care* **2**: 149–50.

Wyatt, J.C. (1994a) Clinical data systems I: data and medical records. *Lancet* **344**: 1543–7.

Wyatt, J.C. (1994b) Clinical data systems II: components and techniques. *Lancet* **344**: 1609–14.

Wyatt, J.C. (1994c) Clinical data systems III: development and evaluation. *Lancet* **344**: 1682–8.

Wyatt, J.C. (1995) Acquisition and use of clinical data for audit and research. *Journal of Evaluation in Clinical Practice* **1**: 15–27.

11 ◆ Clinical Audit and the Availability of Evidence-based Care: The Patient's View

Marianne Rigge

Introduction

Most health professionals are still getting used to the idea of clinical audit. Medical audit advisory groups (MAAGs), responsible for the organisation of audit in primary healthcare, have by and large not yet been replaced by clinical audit advisory groups (CAAGs). Hospital-based clinical audit groups may have been set up, but they often hide the fact that uniprofessional audit continues and is largely dominated by medical audit (Buttery *et al.* 1994). This is hardly surprising. We still inhabit a professional culture which made it acceptable for a 1989 working paper on medical audit to state quite unequivocally that 'the quality of medical work can only be reviewed by a doctor's peers' (1989).

By March 1994, £220 million had been spent on developing clinical audit, the lion's share – £160 million – being spent on medical audit alone. Little wonder that nurses and the professions allied to medicine may lack confidence or feel diffident about playing a major part in the development of clinical audit, though moves to encourage and enhance multidisciplinary audit team work are greatly to be welcomed (Firth-Cozens 1992).

It is not, perhaps, surprising that most patients have never heard of clinical audit and that they would not know what it meant. Even when they are involved in it, to the extent that their medical records and case histories are discussed by doctors, most remain unaware of their involvement in audit (Rigge 1994a). Certainly, most patients will never get to see the results – even if an audit has shown that they received an unacceptable standard of treatment – because results are very rarely published. Nor will they be asked for their views about the outcome of audit. In the worst case scenario, it is patients' solicitors who will get access to their records, prior to taking out a case for medical negligence and this is surely not as it should be.

Far too many patients have a touching faith that the doctor knows best and that the treatment they are being offered is the best available. Most would be shocked to learn how little we actually know about the efficacy of even quite common treatments and procedures, and even more shocked at the variations that exist in outcomes (as Miles *et al.*

discuss in Chapter 1), some of which are quite unacceptable (Buck *et al.* 1987; Campling *et al.* 1990). Even when information about treatments is available, patients experience difficulties with the content and method of communication (Audit Commission 1993). It has also been suggested that a lack of knowledge of health professionals may provide a barrier to giving patients the information they need (Smith *et al.* 1994).

This chapter will give an overview of some of the main issues affecting patients in today's health service, in the light of recent developments in consumerism and the move towards more evidence-based care. It will also consider how clinical guidelines could be made more patient centred.

A decade of change

The past decade has been a time of momentous change in the NHS. My own perspective is that of director of a patient organisation, the College of Health in London, which was set up in 1983. My co-founder, Michael Young – one of the founders of consumerism in the UK – spelt out the reasons for doing so in the first issue of our then journal, *Self Health*.

> 'The reason for establishing the College of Health lies in the present imbalance between medical professionals and their patients. The former have power, the latter do not. This is not just owing to the emotional dependence which many sick people cannot avoid. It is also owing to the large gap between the knowledge and information of the two parties. Information, as always, is power.'
>
> (Rigge 1993.)

The age of the informed consumer?

Times have changed. We have got a Patient's Charter (DoH 1991); the NHS Executive has set up a Patient Empowerment Focus Group; and the Clinical Outcomes Group, chaired by the Chief Medical Officer and the Chief Nursing Officer has set up a consumer subgroup which has recently reported on consumer involvement in clinical audit and outcomes or, rather more to the point, the lack of it (Kelson 1995). There is also a consumer member of the clinical guidelines subgroup, and the Secretary of State has organised a quality initiative culminating in the publication of 'patient perception booklets' aimed at both purchasers and providers (NHSME 1993a; 1994a).

Since 1992, we have also had a nationwide network of health information services with a freephone telephone number, 0800 665544. Any member of the public can ring this number and ask for information about virtually any aspect of the health service and expect to get an answer. My contribution reflects the fact that I have participated in most of these initiatives and so write as what you might call a 'professional consumer'.

A new vocabulary

There is, now, a whole new jargon to accompany these changes. Alongside 'clinical audit', 'meta-analysis' and 'evidence-based care', we have 'shared decision making', 'patient focused care', 'graduated patient care', 'seamless care', 'patient empowerment' and 'user involvement'. What does it all mean? How much of it is rhetoric and how much is reality?

The problem facing patients

The College of Health has built up a wealth of experience in the everyday problems people face in their dealings with the NHS. We have, for example, helped tens of thousands of patients facing unacceptably long waits for hospital treatment through our Guide to Hospital Waiting Lists and National Waiting List Helpline. We currently take some 80 calls a day on our Healthline service, the regional health information service for the former North East Thames Regional Health Authority. The same number of people again call out of hours to listen to one of the nearly 400 pre-recorded tapes on a wide range of health and medical subjects. Over the past 11 years, the tapes most frequently requested have consistently included subjects which people feel embarrassed, nervous or diffident about bothering their doctor with, such as anxiety and depression, irritable bowel syndrome, the menopause and cancer of the colon.

Patients clearly want more information than they are able to get from their doctors (Buckland 1994). They appreciate guidance on what they can do to help themselves, where else they can go for help and advice and, increasingly, what sort of standards of care they should reasonably be able to expect. The Patient's Charter has helped to arouse such expectations but it has so far largely avoided tackling clinical, as opposed to organisational issues. Where clinical issues are dealt with, the things that matter to patients are fudged, for example the Charter sets out the right

> 'to be referred to a consultant acceptable to you, when your GP thinks it necessary, and to be referred for a second opinion if you and your GP agree this is desirable'.
>
> (DoH 1991.)

Leaving aside the problems which arise when patient and GP disagree about the need for a second opinion (especially when the GP is fundholding and will have to pay directly for that opinion), how is any patient to know whether or not a consultant is acceptable to them? How, for that matter, do GPs find out about the qualifications and expertise of surgeons? How much freedom do GPs have, even if they are willing to let patients exercise their choice of consultant? These questions are beginning to be asked publicly by consumer organisations (Rigge 1995), the national press (Rigge 1994a) and even medical publications (Rigge 1994b). Unfortunately, the answers are not so easily forthcoming.

There is no systematic way to get reliable, up-to-date information about centres of expertise or about consultants who specialise within their specialty. There are, however, some promising signs of change. Trust hospitals are beginning to produce glossy brochures for fund-holding GPs and some of these include information on performance indicators and outcomes as well as price. The Cancer Relief Macmillan Fund recently published a directory of breast cancer services in the UK (CRMF 1995), though it did not include the names of the dedicated breast cancer surgeons who work within them. Nevertheless, it is a welcome step in the right direction.

Another welcome step is the recent publication of the Department of Health's code of practice on openness which suggests that Trusts should make available information about the qualifications and areas of special interests of their clinicians (NHSME 1995). The support of the medical profession is to some extent given implicit recognition by a recent statement from the Royal Surgical Colleges of Great Britain and Ireland which states that

> 'a surgeon who performs a specific operation once or twice a year is unlikely to be as experienced, and therefore as competent, as a surgeon who performs the same procedure 30 times a year'.
> (Royal Surgical Colleges 1994.)

They say that very rare conditions should be treated, and the rarest operations carried out, only in specialist centres of expertise. Unfortunately, the Colleges fail to suggest which conditions or operations these might be, nor do they identify the centres of expertise. No such lists have been published, either by the Royal Colleges or by the Department of Health.

In the meantime, experience at the College of Health suggests that doctors do not always know best, nor that they are necessarily able to do the best they could for their patients as the following examples show.

A woman wrote to the college in 1994 about two problems, both of them affecting her adult children. This was not an articulate, middle class parent insisting on special treatment; she was simply a caring mother who could see that things were not right. Her daughter, who had a gynaecological complaint and was a virgin, had previously been mortified by the treatment she received from a male doctor and was adamant that she would only be seen by a female doctor. Unfortunately, all the consultants at their local hospital were male and, as the GP was not fundholding, he could not refer to one of the specialist women's hospitals. That need not necessarily have mattered because most consultants nowadays have at least one woman junior doctor on their firm and, on ringing the medical secretaries, the College of Health discovered that this was indeed the case for the consultant in question. However, the length of the waiting list was such that there would be a new set of junior doctors by the time the patient had her appointment in 1995 and so there was no guarantee that she could be seen by a woman.

The woman's son had a more serious problem. He had been attacked in his home in 1992 by burglars, who had tied him up and stood on his shoulders and neck. As a result, both this young man's shoulders were constantly dislocating; he was having fits, was in great pain and in danger of losing his job. He and his mother were most alarmed when the local hospital doctor said that he would have to look up the treatment that would be called for. The doctor then asked his patient to return in several months time; hardly the sort of thing to inspire you with confidence and hence the mother's letter to the College of Health.

In the circumstances, we suggested she asked the GP to refer her son for a second opinion from the consultant who runs the shoulder unit at one of the specialist orthopaedic hospitals. The local hospital did not feel this necessary. The family were told that a new doctor was arriving soon, one who had been trained at an orthopaedic hospital (though not necessarily in the treatment of dislocating shoulders, as we realised). The appointment was again deferred and an extra contractual referral (ECR) was discouraged. With support from the College of Health and the agreement of the GP, the mother and son persisted and the son was eventually seen in out-patients at the specialist hospital. There, it was agreed that he needed a bilateral shoulder reconstruction and that the operation must be done by the consultant himself.

Unfortunately, by April 1995 the son was still on the waiting list and had been told that it might be another year before he could have his operation. Since it had taken so long for the ECR to be approved, this extended wait was within the letter, if not the spirit, of the Patient's Charter. At least the patient knows that this major operation will be carried out by a consultant who specialises within his specialty. Not all patients are so lucky.

Second class treatment

Patients neither want, nor deserve, second class treatment. But all too often, this is what they get. A recent Cancer Relief Macmillan Fund study found that fewer than half the 30 000 women diagnosed with breast cancer each year ever get to see a consultant who specialises in their condition (CRMF 1994).

What that means in practice, is that some women will die perhaps needlessly. One of these, whose solicitor got in touch with the College of Health earlier this year, was seen by a general surgeon whose specialty is urology. When she asked him about adjuvant treatment and breast reconstruction, he told her that he did not take kindly to patients telling him what to do after reading articles in women's magazines. When she complained, the hospital's medical director said, 'I know – but we can't tell them what to do' (Rigge 1995). At the time of writing she has months to live.

The need for patient-centred guidelines

Patients would not need to rely on women's magazines for information about their illnesses or to know what questions to ask the doctor if they had access to decent guidelines about the treatment they should properly expect.

The current uncertainty about how guidelines should be produced, by whom and for whom, is unhelpful to say the least. Few have been endorsed nationally, though a start has been made with the setting up of a clinical guidelines subgroup of the Clinical Outcomes Group and its early work has resulted in some national guidance for purchasers and providers (NHSME 1993b, 1994b). The Royal Colleges and other professional bodies are anxious about the legal implications of clinical guidelines which Hurwitz, writing in Chapter 9, has elegantly discussed. Perhaps understandably, they are proceeding with caution, producing in some cases only one or two sets of guidelines a year. This is not much help to patients who need guidance now about current good practice for even very common conditions, let alone those that are rare.

When considered in this light, the over-cautious approach that is taken, either for fear of litigation or out of an excessive regard for the sanctity of clinical freedom, is perhaps misplaced. In fact, it could be argued that, as far as litigation is concerned, the opening up of information to patients about risks and alternatives means rather that they will take a much greater share in the responsibility for decisions they and their doctors jointly take. As for the threats to clinical freedom and innovation that are commonly invoked when discussing guidelines, you have only to look at the positive, perhaps even over-positive response of patients to developments in minimal access therapy, to see that they are anything but a threat to innovation. Indeed, when it comes to new treatments for chronic or incurable illness, there are probably far more patients who would like to be offered the chance of trying these than are ever actually involved in clinical trials. Patients who know they are likely to die sooner rather than later may have little patience with the arguments for proceeding slowly and with caution when it can take so many years to produce the results of randomised controlled trials that are needed for evidence based care.

A definition of guidelines

What can guidelines possibly be but guides? The Chief Medical Officer, Kenneth Calman, gave a most helpful description at a meeting of the Clinical Outcomes Group held in London in February 1995:

'Clinical guidelines are an aid to good clinical practice. They should improve the way patients are cared for, reduce unacceptable and inappropriate variations, and improve outcomes. They are not an end in themselves.'

The very term 'guidelines' suggests, at any rate to a layman, that they are something you steer by. If an unexpected side effect or co-morbidity presents itself, you alter your course. Patients know this, for they are individuals with their own hopes, fears, likes, dislikes, experiences and views.

It follows that patients and, where appropriate, their carers, should be involved in the planning, development, implementation, monitoring and evaluation of clinical guidelines. They should also be involved in the ensuing development and implementation of the clinical audit protocols which should, as Anthony Hopkins has recently pointed out, be an integral part of the guidelines development process (Hopkins 1995). That is not to say that patients will not need to be better educated and informed, nor that consumer representatives, where these are invited to be involved in the processes of clinical audit, will not need training and support.

Taking account of qualitative research

Reviews of the literature, both published and unpublished, should include reviews of qualitative research into patients' views of the process and outcome of treatment. An example of this research is the consumer audit studies carried out by the College of Health using in-depth interviews and focus group discussions to find out patients' views and experiences of the process and outcome of treatment (CoH 1994).

The remit given to guideline committees should stress the need to consider the whole experience of the patient, throughout the course of their diagnosis, treatment and recovery. Put simply, this would mean saying 'If your parent or spouse or child were suffering from this condition, what would you like to happen to them from the point at which they developed symptoms through to a successful recovery, or palliative care, as the case may be?'

Towards more patient-centred guidelines

The implications of this are that patient-centred guidelines should include the following:

(1) Referral protocols, to encourage GPs to make timely and appropriate referrals.

(2) Agreement about what diagnostic and other tests should be ordered, by whom, and at what stage – as well as how, when and by whom the results should be communicated to patients.

(3) Where appropriate, protocols for pain relief and other symptom management should also be agreed, especially for those patients unable to take analgesics, for example because they have developed gastric ulcers, hiatus hernias or other conditions related to their prolonged use of prescribed painkillers.

(4)   Awareness of the need to guide patients towards sources of information, help and advice for coping with their illness and its effects, especially if they have to wait for extended periods before treatment can be carried out. This might include physiotherapy and occupational therapy, aids and adaptations available through social services, welfare and other benefits, and self help groups and voluntary organisations of which there are at least 1400 nationally.

(5)   Awareness of the fact that many conditions – and many patients – do not present with a single, clear-cut condition or diagnosis. Many illnesses are multi-factorial in causation and presentation; some may not ever be satisfactorily diagnosed. That is not to say that patients do not need the best standards of treatment and management of the uncertainty which can be as distressing for them as for their clinicians.

(6)   Discharge protocols to ensure that patients receive the full range of information, advice and support when they are sent out from hospital, as set out above.

Information to patients about guidelines

It should be standard practice for clinical guidelines committees to produce a patient version – as is commonplace in the USA – in which medical terminology is explained in lay terms. This is already the case for those involved in carrying out research trials where patients are required to give informed consent. It is perhaps a discipline for which some clinicians may need training in communication skills.

The group on guidelines for the management of women with adverse effects following radiotherapy for breast cancer, which has recently submitted its report to the Chief Medical Officer and the Clinical Outcomes Groups, provides an admirable example of how this might be achieved (Maher 1995). This had no token consumer representative. Instead six patient organisations – BACUP, Cancerlink, Breast Cancer Care, the Patients' Association, the College of Health and, most importantly, a group of women who have actually suffered long-term serious adverse effects following radiotherapy for breast cancer – were represented alongside all the different health professionals involved in the treatment and care of such patients. It is these consumer groups which are currently working together to produce patient information leaflets based on the guidelines.

An educative and constructive process

In general, patients who are well informed about good practice are much more likely to report back in a positive, informative and constructive way on outcomes and on whether or not guidelines have been followed. This should be an intrinsic part of clinical audit. Indeed the very act of asking well-informed questions about treatment choices based on acknowledged good practice, could be educative for doctors and result in better adherence to guidelines unless there are good reasons not to.

Over-reliance on science

A rigid insistence that guidelines must be based on the evidence of scientific trials may be unhelpful to patients. Medicine is an art as well as a science and sometimes results will depend as much on patient compliance as on the treatment administered. This, in turn, may depend on the quality of communication with patients and that of the information they are given.

Taken to its logical conclusion, an insistence that guidelines should only be based on the results of randomised controlled trials would mean that it would be impossible to produce guidelines for many surgical procedures, including the majority of the new minimally invasive procedures, since virtually none of these has been the subject of controlled trials. It also begs a number of questions about the size and quality of some trials and the fact that there is a bias towards reporting only those that have been successful. In real life, most people learn rather more from their failures than from their successes.

It is clearly in everyone's interests to encourage the development of evidence-based medicine, but this must be done in the context both of medical and scientific uncertainty and of the uniqueness of every transaction that takes place between doctors and their patients. Caution must therefore be exercised in the 'buying' of protocols of care, as Miles *et al.* emphasise in Chapter 8 of this volume. We need to recognise the real needs of those patients for whom diagnosis has not proved possible and those for whom, despite a diagnosis, there is no effective treatment. The needs are especially great when the patients' problems have in fact been caused by the treatment they have received, as in the case of the women who suffered long-term adverse effects from radiotherapy following breast cancer. As the secretary of the British Medical Association has recently said:

'The challenge is to promote the practice of evidence-based medicine without imposing a defensive paralysis on the profession.'

(Armstrong 1995.)

Conclusion

At the present rate of guideline development, we are many years away from being able to tell patients suffering from even the most common conditions, what sort of standard of treatment they should be able to expect. Where there is confusion and uncertainty, they deserve to be told that. What is needed is a more pragmatic and patient-centred approach.

References

Armstrong, M. (1995) We must not let science bind us, *BMA News Review*, March.

Audit Commission (1993) *What Seems to be the Matter? Communication Between Hospitals and Patients*, HMSO London.

Buck, N., Devlin, H.B. & Lunn, J.N. (1987) *The Report of the Confidential Enquiry into Perioperative Deaths*, Nuffield Provincial Hospitals Trust and the King Edward's Hospital Fund for London, London.

Buckland, S. (1994) Unmet needs for health information: a literature review. *Health Libraries Review* **11**: 82–9.

Buttery, Y., Walshe, K., Coles, J. & Bennett, J. (1994) *Evaluating Medical Audit: The Development of Audit – Findings of a National Survey of Healthcare, Provider Units in England*, CASPE Research, London.

Campling, E.A., Devlin, H.B. & Lunn, J.N. (1990) *The Report of the National Confidential Enquiry into Perioperative Deaths 1989*, NCEPOD, London.

CoH (1994) *Consumer Audit Guidelines*, College of Health, London.

CRMF (1994) *The Macmillan Prima Breast Cancer Survey*, Cancer Relief Macmillan Fund, London.

CRMF (1995) *Macmillan Director of Breast Cancer Services in the UK*, Cancer Relief Macmillan Fund, London.

DoH (1989) *Working for Patients*, HMSO, London.

DoH (1991) *Patient's Charter*, Department of Health, HMSO, London.

Firth-Cozens, I.J. (1992) Building teams for effective audit. *Quality in Health Care* **1**: 151–5.

Hopkins, A. (1995) Some reservations about clinical guidelines. *Archives of Disease in Childhood* **72**: 70–5.

Kelson, M. (1995) *Consumer Involvement Initiatives in Clinical Audit and Outcomes: A Review of Developments and Issues in the Identification of Good Practice*, College of Health, London.

Maher, E.J. (1995) *Report of Group on Guidelines for Management of Women with Adverse Effects following Breast Radiotherapy*, Royal College of Radiologists, London.

NHSME (1993a) *Patient Perception Booklet Series*, NHS Management Executive, Department of Health, Leeds.

NHSME (1993b) *Improving Clinical Effectiveness*, EL(93)115, NHS Management Executive, Department of Health, Leeds.

NHSME (1994a) *Patient Perception Booklet Series*, National Health Service Management Executive, Department of Health, Leeds.

NHSME (1994b), *Improving the Effectiveness of the NHS*, EL(194)74, NHS Management Executive, Department of Health, Leeds.

NHSME (1995) *Code of Practice on Openness in the NHS*, NHS Management Executive, Department of Health, Leeds.

Rigge, M. (1993) Involving patients and consumers. *Health Service Journal Management Guide*, September.

Rigge, M. (1994a) Involving patients in clinical audit. *Quality in Health Care* **3** (Suppl.): S3–S5.

Rigge, M. (1994b) The patient's dilemma, *The Guardian*, 23 November, p. 14.

Rigge, M. (1994c) Whose outcome is it anyway? In: *Outcomes Into Clinical Care* (ed. T. Delamothe) BMJ Press, London.

Rigge, M. (1995) *Which doctor?* Which? *Way to Health*, Consumers' Association, London.

Royal Surgical Colleges (1994) *Quality Assurance: The Role of Training, Certification, Audit and Continuing Professional Education in the Maintenance of the Highest Possible Standards of Clinical Practice*, Senate of the Royal Surgical Colleges of Great Britain and Ireland, London.
Smith, D. *et al.* (1994) Lack of knowledge in health professionals: a barrier to providing information to patients. *Quality in Health Care* **3**: 75–8.

Appendix
Available Information on Clinical Effectiveness

Institutions

(1) NHS centre for Reviews and Dissemination (CRD). Database of published reviews, economic evaluation and commissions reviews available on disk. For further details contact:
   NHS Centre for Review & Dissemination
   University of York
   Heslington
   York YO1 5DD

(2) Outcomes Clearing House publishes regular Outcomes Briefing and promotes advice on outcome measures to the NHS. For further details contact:
   UK Clearing House on Health Outcomes
   Nuffield Institute
   71–5 Clarendon Road
   Leeds LS2 9PL

Documents

(1) *Effective Healthcare Bulletin* is published regularly, covering issues such as screening for osteoporosis, stroke rehabilitation, glue ear, depression in primary care and subfertility. For further details contact:
   Effective Health Care
   Nuffield Institute for Health
   71–5 Clarendon Road
   Leeds LS2 9PL

(2) The Cochrane databases of systematic reviews are regularly updated and evaluated from the BMJ publishing group. For further details contact:
   UK Cochrane Centre
   Summertown Pavilion
   Middle Way
   Oxford OX2 7LG

(3) Health of the Nation Target Effectiveness Documents, e.g. Target

effectiveness and cost effectiveness guide for CHD/stroke. For further details contact:
Department of Health
80 London Road
Elephant and Castle
London SE1 6LW

(4) Confidential Enquiries Reports, including:

- *Still Births and Death in Infancy*
- *Maternal Deaths*
- *Perioperative and Operative Deaths*
- *Counselling for Genetic Disorders.*

For further details contact:
Department of Health
80 London Road
Elephant and Castle
London SE1 6LW

(5) Health of the Nation key area handbooks

(6) Epidemiologically based needs assessment covering topics such as diabetes mellitus, hip and knee replacement, strokes, renal discose, hernia repair. For further details contact:
NHS Executive
Quarry House
Quarry Hill
Leeds LS2 7UE

Index